Computing and information management in general practice

Peter Schattner

SECOND EDITION

The *McGraw·Hill* Companies

Sydney New York San Francisco Auckland
Bangkok Bogotá Caracas Hong Kong
Kuala Lumpur Lisbon London Madrid
Mexico City Milan New Delhi San Juan
Seoul Singapore Taipei Toronto

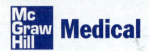

First published by McGraw-Hill 2007

Text © 2007 Peter Schattner and the Royal Australian College of General Practitioners
Illustrations and design © 2007 McGraw-Hill Australia Pty Ltd
Additional owners of copyright are acknowledged on the Acknowledgments page.

National Library of Australia Cataloguing-in-Publication data:
Schattner, Peter.
    Computing and information management in general practice.

    2nd ed.
    Includes index.
    ISBN 9780074717776.

    1. Medicine - Data processing. 2. Medical offices -
    Management - Data processing. 3. Computers. I. Title.

610.285

Published in Australia by
McGraw-Hill Australia Pty Ltd
Level 2, 82 Waterloo Road, North Ryde NSW 2113
Publisher: Nicole Meehan
Managing Editor: Jo Munnelly
Production Editor: Samantha Miles
Editor: Leanne Poll
Manager, Rights and Permissions: Jared Dunn
Designer (cover and interior): Robert Klinkhamer
Typeset in Helvetica Neue by Kim Webber
Proofreader: Kathryn Murphy
Illustrations: Ian F Faulkner & Associates
Indexer: Madeleine Davis
Printed in China on 90 gsm woodfree by CTPS

Foreword

Over the past decade Australian general practice has embraced the use of computers to support improvements in the safety and quality of care provided to our patients. We know that the majority of Australia's general practitioners are now using computerised medical record systems to enter and store the details of patient consultations and that most are using a computer for key tasks such as prescribing, recording allergies, ordering laboratory tests, receiving results and writing referrals to consultant specialists.

In a set of clear and concise chapters, Professor Peter Schattner has produced an excellent primer for all those who work in general practice in Australia on the safe and appropriate use of computers.

The book has been written with the busy practitioner in mind. It includes checklists, warnings, reminders, case studies, practical exercises and a lot of commonsense advice to assist you to get the most out of the clinical system in your practice. It focuses on the growing use of the Internet in medical practice and the rise in the use of clinical decision support systems that can support doctors and nurses in the daily care of their patients. The book also has a special focus on how we can work in partnership with our patients to use this new technology to support their individual care.

If implemented, the lessons in this book have the potential to support significant improvements in the standards of general practice care provided to the people of Australia. While information technology can change rapidly over a short time, many of the basic principles outlined in this book should continue to be relevant into the future.

I commend this book to everyone who is concerned about ensuring that computers are used in a way that supports safe, high-quality general practice care. This book will be of interest to general practitioners, general practice nurses, practice managers and receptionists, staff of Divisions of General Practice and members of professional organisations committed to standards and quality care. It will also be a valuable resource for computer science students and researchers who are seeking to understand the context of general practice and the challenge of computerising a complex distributed system of health care delivery. And I also expect that many consumers of health care will be fascinated to learn how their own local general practice is using information technology to support improvements in the care provided to individual patients and the wider community.

Professor Michael Kidd
Head of the Discipline of General Practice at the University of Sydney
Inaugural chair of the Australian General Practice Computing Group (1997–2002)
President of The Royal Australian College of General Practitioners (2002–2006)

Contents

CHAPTER TWO
Computers and practice management p22

02

CONTENTS

CHAPTER THREE

Computers and clinical care p42

03

04

CHAPTER FIVE

Computer security and general practice   p90

05

CHAPTER SIX

Promoting quality and safety in GP computing   p110

06

Preface

This book comprises a set of comprehensive educational resources which provide practical information on how to make the best use of computers in general practice. The resources cover clinical and administrative uses of computers, provide tips for enhancing computer security, and raise some legal, ethical and quality issues for consideration.

Although written in Australia, the principles outlined in this book should be relevant to other countries that are at a similar stage of computerisation of general practice. The advice has not been written with specific software packages in mind and can be used for a variety of them, both here and overseas.

The book can be used by general practitioners (GPs), GP registrars and general practice staff as stand-alone resources, but will also be useful for divisions of general practice and other professional organisations as support material for their own information management and information technology (IM/IT) educational programs. It is written in such a way that technical expertise is not required to understand and use the suggestions made.

Mention of particular software packages or websites is not meant as an endorsement of any one product over another. These are simply used as examples. The book is also not intended to replace guidelines provided in other publications, such as the RACGP *Standards for General Practices*, or the many worthwhile resources produced by divisions of general practice and others.

Obviously, GPs vary in their computer skills. Some parts of the text will therefore seem 'basic' to those with more experience; it might at times be fairly advanced for others. Overall, it is aimed at the middle ground.

The main part of the book is arranged into five separate chapters which are of particular relevance to GPs, trainees and practice staff. The topics are:
- issues concerning the triad of computers, GPs and patients
- using computers for practice management
- using computers for clinical care
- using electronic resources, especially the Internet, for clinical purposes
- computer security.

The final chapter takes a bigger-picture view of the promotion of quality and safety in the use of computers by GPs. This includes a guide for divisions of general practice as well as suggestions for government, GP organisations and the medical software industry.

Finally, a word on terminology. This book refers to the word 'computing' and 'information management' rather than informatics or other descriptive terms. The reason is that we are mainly interested in the day-to-day use of computers by GPs and not a theoretical understanding of information science or computer science. 'Computing' seems a reasonable choice to highlight that this book is about GPs using computers to improve the health of patients and to run practices more efficiently through effective use of information.

Peter Schattner

Acknowledgments

This book is based on a series of educational modules produced under the auspices of the General Practice Computing Group (GPCG). The chapters in this book are the direct counterparts of the original modules. The following authors made major contributions to the earlier modules in the series:

- Module 1 (Computers, GPs and patients): Hester Gascoigne and Bob Milstein
- Module 2 (Clinical care): Dr Trevor Lord
- Module 3 (Practice management): Paul Zucker
- Module 4 (Electronic resources): Associate Professor Peter Schattner and Dr Ken Harvey
- Module 5 (Computer security): Associate Professor Peter Schattner
- Module 6 (A guide for divisions of general practice): Ms Leonie Harrison.

The following members of the GPCG Quality Care Delivery Working Group and the GPCG Consumer Reference Group (CRG) are acknowledged for their review of and input into the original modules: Dr Oliver Frank, Ms Catherine Pleteschner, Ms Dell Horey, Ms Diane Walsh, Dr Trevor Lord, Professor Michael Kidd, Ms Jan Donovan and Mr David Camus.

Individual contributors on behalf of the GPCG were:

- Ms Marta Veroni, Editor
- Dr Ronald McCoy
- Dr Chris Pearce
- Dr Louise McCall, learning objectives
- Dr John Togno, input regarding the legal issues in Module 1.

Ms Leonie Harrison, as the GPCG Project Officer, made a very substantial contribution to the 'module project' by managing the enterprise, making suggestions to authors and by contributing in no small way to the written materials. She ably supported the project leader, Peter Schattner.

Other organisations involved with the original modules were:

- the Australian General Practice Network (formerly the Australian Divisions of General Practice)
- state-based organisations (SBOs)

- the Australian Department of Health and Ageing, which provided support and funding.

The Royal Australian College of General Practitioners (RACGP) has provided considerable assistance in the creation of this book. Various people have commented on drafts of some of the chapters, including Ms Mary Mathews and Mr John Feore from the Monash Division of General Practice and Ms Teri Snowden from the RACGP.

About the principal author

Peter Schattner is a GP in Melbourne and a part-time clinical associate professor in the department of general practice, Monash University. He is also the IM/IT adviser to the Monash Division of General Practice.

He has 20 years' experience in primary care health services research and is involved in post-graduate distance education. He has a longstanding interest in general practice computing and has conducted a number of national consultancies and research projects in this field.

As principal author, Peter has revised and updated the original materials, which were, in part, written by others.

He is supported by a tolerant wife and three young adult children. When the home computer crashes, they know not to call him.

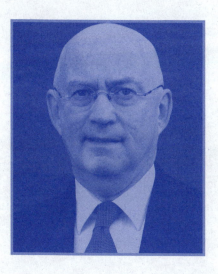

Computers, GPs and patients: issues in general practice

This chapter considers the use and impact of information management (IM) and information technology (IT) in general practice, and how to make best use of computers in the consultation. This chapter also discusses privacy and confidentiality of consumer health information, and provides an overview of related legal issues.

CONTENTS

When you have completed this chapter, you will be able to:

- gain increased benefit from the use of computers within the consultation

---

- provide patients with information about the use of computers within the practice

---

- communicate with your patients by email in a clinically responsible and safe manner

---

- understand consumer concerns about the use of computers in general practice

---

- describe consumers' rights in relation to their electronic health information, including their rights to access and privacy

---

- understand your obligations when transferring electronic information to third parties, such as other health care providers

---

- manage patient information within a legal and ethical framework

---

- assess medicolegal risks of using computers in general practice.

Introduction

This book sets out to support general practice computing in a number of ways. First, it provides general practitioners (GPs) with guidelines and tips on how to use computers in a number of distinct areas, from practice administration to clinical computing and use of the Internet. Second, it is a useful resource for those who wish to support and train GPs and general practice staff on the use of computers. It can therefore be used, for example, by divisions of general practice. Third, it attempts to set out standards for general practice computing, so that GPs have a benchmark of what they might be expected to know and be skilled at.

The chapters in this book cover the use of computers from several perspectives. The first chapter is largely about the doctor–patient–computer relationship. This is a good place to start, as the patient is the real reason why standards in general practice computing are so important. There is reasonable evidence now that computers can assist in better patient care. This is especially so in medication management, but has also been shown across several other clinical domains. A brief background on computer usage and policy developments is provided first.

Background

The relatively recent uptake of computers in Australian general practice has been mirrored in many other countries. Surveys in Australia reveal that approximately 15 per cent of GPs used computers in their practices in 1997. This had risen to 70 per cent by the year 2000, and 90 per cent by 2005.

Why did this happen? There are likely to be several reasons for this, including the following:

- Direct financial incentives to GPs through the government-funded Practice Incentives Program. From 1998, GPs could claim grants in addition to their fee-for-service income if they met certain criteria, several of which related to the use of computers.
- The development of cheap and well-customised clinical software. One of the main packages sent to GPs free of charge was subsidised by pharmaceutical companies that provided advertisements which popped up during program use. Clearly, GPs were 'ready' to use a reasonably intuitive program that at the very least made prescribing easier.
- Training and support for GPs. Divisions of General Practice, which are regional support organisations funded by the Australian Government, ran an 'IT officer program' between 1999 and 2001. The IT officers provided a variety of training opportunities for GPs, and in some cases, fulfilled a 'helpdesk' role for practices that were having trouble with their hardware or software.
- GP leadership in IT within the medical profession. The Australian Government also funded the General Practice Computing Group (GPCG) between 1998 and 2005. The GPCG provided a leadership role in general practice computing, helping to set standards, overseeing the IT officer program and commissioning a number of projects to examine aspects of GP computing in detail. It helped bring general practice to the forefront of computing within the broader medical profession.

These factors were probably the main reasons why there was a relatively rapid uptake of computers for both administrative and clinical tasks in general practice within the space of a few years. Most recent studies have shown that while virtually all GPs who use computers for clinical purposes use them for prescribing, other areas are lagging behind (see Table 1.1).

**TABLE 1.1 CLINICAL USE OF COMPUTERS BY AUSTRALIAN GPs IN 2005
(AS % OF GPS WITH COMPUTERS IN CONSULTING ROOMS)**

- Prescribing (98%)
- Order laboratory test (using printed form) (85%)
- Record drug allergies (84%)
- General health summaries (84%)
- Write referral letters (81%)
- Receive pathology results via electronic download (79%)
- Run recall system (e.g. Pap tests) (77%)
- Chronic or complex disease management plan (e.g. diabetes) (68%)
- Record progress notes (64%)
- Access patient education material (63%)
- Conduct clinical audits (56%)

- Internet use (67%)
- Email use (59%)

Source: D. Keith McInnes, Deborah C. Saltman and Michael R. Kidd, 2006, 'General practitioners' use of computers for prescribing and electronic health records: results from a national survey', *Medical Journal of Australia*, 185 (2): 88–91

Unfortunately, ongoing training and support has become quite patchy, although recently the Australian Government agreed to fund a Regional Health Information Management Officers (RHIMO) program. RHIMOs work with divisions but operate at the level of the divisions' state-based organisations. The program is being given direction at the national level through the Australian General Practice Network (AGPN).

Table 1.1 is also revealing in that electronic communication with hospitals, medical specialists and allied health professionals does not appear to be a common GP task. Although the government set up the National E-Health Transition Authority (NEHTA, see **www.nehta.gov.au**) to develop a standards framework for computing across the whole health spectrum, this remains a work in progress, with little implementation on the ground.

Patient focus

So, let us start with patients, and fit GPs and computers around them. This approach will make you appreciate:

- the benefits and drawbacks of using computers in the consultation
- patient rights and GP obligations
- maximising the benefits and minimising the risks of using computers in the consultation.

You should not get overly concerned with medicolegal risk in the computer age. The risk to you has not changed all that much. Effective computer use supports good patient care and the efficient running of the practice, and is therefore simply in everyone's best interest.

Computers and the consultation

It is rare nowadays to find a GP who does not have a computer on his or her desk, but not all GPs have the same level of skill or use computers in the same way.

Most GPs use a computer to write prescriptions, request tests and view test results. Some also use a computer to record immunisations, create health summaries and write referrals. Some GPs extend their computer usage to create care plans and share information with other health professionals.

Used well, the computer can help you plan and keep track of your patient's health care. Compared with paper-based records, computers can make it easier and quicker to:

- find a patient's health information when you need it
- read the information—electronic records are more legible than handwritten notes
- check medications and test results
- make referrals
- keep track of follow-ups, reminders and screening checks
- share and discuss information with your patients
- share information with other health professionals
- provide alerts for potential problems such as adverse drug reactions or interactions.

The advice that follows might seem obvious, especially to experienced GPs. However, research has shown that many GPs remain uncomfortable with the new GP–patient–computer triad. In part, this is because GPs with insufficient keyboard skills are 'peckers' rather than confident typists. Too much concentration on which key to press and what to do next with the computer program can divert your attention from your patients during the consultation.

This chapter, and those that follow, provide some commonsense advice that should help you improve your computer skills so that the technology assists rather than hinders patient care.

CAN THE DOCTOR–PATIENT RELATIONSHIP WORK IN A COMPUTERISED WORLD?

Doctors will each use computers in different ways, just as doctors vary in their consultation styles. Some type constantly on the computer keyboard. Some alternate between the computer and the patient. Others make handwritten notes for some consultations, such as home visits, and add them to the computer record later.

Not all patients will respond to the computer in the same way. Some will be more computer literate than others. Some may have no interest in what information is stored in the computer. Others may ask to see information (such as test results) in their electronic record. They may ask directly or give a visual cue such as leaning forward to see the results on the screen.

The trick is to find a way to make the computer work for you and your patients. Experiment with different approaches. If in doubt about how to proceed, take your cue from the patient.

REMEMBER!

The computer can help to improve the quality of health care you provide, but it's only a tool. It is not meant to replace the relationship between you and your patients.

HOW CAN I MAKE THE MOST OF THE COMPUTER IN THE CONSULTATION?

The following are tips to make the most of the computer:
- Be confident and competent in using the technology. You don't have to be a touch typist but you do need to understand the features of the program you use.
- Be comfortable with your level of skill rather than embarrassed. Patients don't expect you to be a technology whiz.
- Explain what you are doing. For example, 'I'm just typing a letter to your specialist' or 'I'm ordering some blood tests'.
- Listen to what your patient is saying. Important information is often given as an aside. Don't miss the clues because you're distracted by the computer.

REMEMBER!

However you use your computer, do so in such a way that the patient remains the focus of the consultation.

WHAT DO I NEED TO KNOW ABOUT THE PRIVACY OF PATIENT HEALTH INFORMATION?

As a GP, you generally hold more information about a patient's health than any other individual health care provider.

Most of the time you will be the only one who needs to see that information. However, sometimes a patient's health care plan will require other people to view some or all of a patient's health record. This may

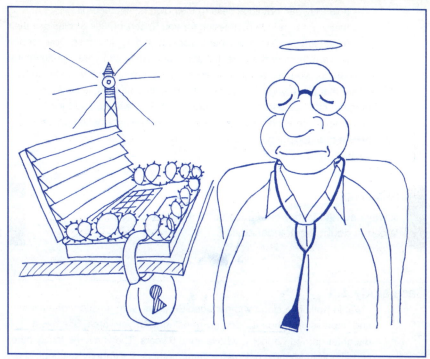

You should take steps to protect the privacy of your patients

include practice nurses, other GPs in your practice or other health professionals outside your practice.

Administration and reception staff generally should not have access to the clinical record. However, they will need to access the computer system to manage bookings and accounts, and view any messages that need to be passed on between patients and doctors.

Patient health information is personal and private and you need to take steps to ensure it stays that way:

- Make sure routine access to a medical record is on a need-to-know basis.
- Use passwords to ensure only the right people see the information.
- Clear the screen after each visit so that one patient cannot see another's record.
- Provide clear written information, such as a waiting room poster or brochure, that explains to patients:
  - how their health information will be stored within the practice
  - who typically has access to it, both within and outside the practice
  - how information is generally transferred to third parties
  - how that information is typically used (e.g. shared care, accreditation, research)

– how they can obtain access to their own health records
– their right to refuse permission for you to collect, use or disclose their health information in any particular way. If they do refuse, you need to warn them of the potential effect on their health care management.

Whether you use a paper or electronic record system, you should be aware that privacy law in Australia, as in other countries, is based on a range of statutes and other legal principles. These laws, and their interaction with each other, can be complex. The information provided here is of a general nature only and is not intended to stand as legal advice.

> **REMEMBER!**
> Always adhere to the principles set out in privacy legislation. When in doubt, seek legal advice.

Case study **1.1**

Melanie Kolly is a single mother aged 28 years, with a history of anxiety and depression, who has recently transferred to your area. She has a daughter named Kimberly, who is aged 6 years. They have no family here, and although Melanie has met several mothers at Kimberly's school, she has not made any close friends.

Melanie sees you for the first time and asks whether the previous clinic has transferred her medical records to you. You reply that the paper file was sent promptly by the previous clinic soon after she requested them to do so. You therefore have a reasonably complete set of medical records in front of you.

You tell Melanie your practice is about to go paperless and you will summarise the transferred medical history onto the computer. She is concerned this means it will be easier for people other than you to gain access to her medical record. She doesn't want the practice staff to know about her depression and doesn't want to run the risk of any of the other mothers finding out until she is ready to tell them.

1 How do you reassure Melanie about the privacy and confidentiality of her electronic record?
2 What additional precautions do you need to take to ensure the electronic record remains private and secure?
3 How might you involve Melanie in the review of her electronic record?

The way you collect and share information about patients is increasingly governed by privacy legislation.

The spirit and the letter of these laws emphasise the importance of a shared understanding between you and your patients, in broad terms, of how and why their information will be used and shared with others. To reach that understanding:

- provide standard information leaflets describing your approach to privacy
- discuss privacy concerns with your patients.

Generally, privacy laws do not stop you from providing team-based care where appropriate, but you must always be mindful not to exceed your patient's expectations.

Always check with the patient before using or sharing their information, especially if you feel it is in a way or for a purpose that they may not expect. To protect your patients' privacy when sharing their information:

- generally de-identify personal health information for research studies and practice audits
- include only necessary and relevant information.

The Australian Government's Enhanced Primary Care program explicitly advises GPs to obtain input from other health care providers on 'careplans' for patients with complex or chronic diseases. This is in order to develop a 'team care arrangement'. The principles of privacy need to be considered when sharing patient health information in this way. Obviously, this applies equally to paper-based and electronic health records.

Case study **1.2**

Melanie is not coping too well at the moment and is concerned about the effect her condition might be having on her daughter. It's been about 12 months since Melanie received any counselling and you suggest that it might be a good idea for her to see one of the psychologists at the local community health centre. You explain you can send details of her health record via fax or email.

1 How much do you tell Melanie about the referral?
2 What precautions do you need to take to ensure the right person receives the information?
3 How would you send the referral electronically?

HOW SAFE IS THE ELECTRONIC RECORD?

Your patients' health information is there when you need it. It can be shared at the touch of a button. But you also know about computer 'crashes', hackers and other ways of losing data. So, how safe is the patient health record in your hands?

There are no foolproof methods to protect information, but with care and good procedures, electronic health records can be safer than paper records.

You need to:

- develop policies for your practice on ethical procedures in relation to the management of confidential personal health information
- make backups (copies) of the health records and store them securely off-site
- use software to protect against viruses and other computer threats.

The patient health record is not only a tool to aid your memory, patients are also entitled to have reasonable expectations of the electronic medical record.

A detailed review of security of patient information can be found in Chapter 5.

REMEMBER!

You hold confidential and sensitive information about patients. Make sure you take all reasonable steps to ensure it stays private and secure.

WHAT IS eCONSULTING?

An emerging form of medical practice in the computer age is online consulting. This means that patients can, for a fee, obtain medical advice from registered medical practitioners through the Internet. There are a number of sites which offer this service. Obviously, advice can only be based on the patient's symptoms or description of their problem, and these services are unlikely to put traditional, face-to-face medical practice out of business. However, they might be a way of obtaining expert national or international advice on specific medical problems.

Most of this will not be relevant to your medical practice. As it carries its own particular risks of misdiagnosis, inappropriate advice or misunderstanding by the patient, you might think it better to leave eConsulting to the 'entrepreneurs' at this stage. However, you will be more likely to offer a limited email service, as explained on the following page.

Communicating with your patients by email

WHAT IF MY PATIENTS WANT TO COMMUNICATE WITH ME BY EMAIL?

When your patients need to see you, they make an appointment and attend the practice at the agreed time.

But what if a patient doesn't actually need to 'see' you?

There are times when they may simply want to ask a question such as, 'Do you have the results of my blood tests?' or 'I've lost my prescription—can you write me another one?'.

You and your patient may agree to monitor some aspects of their health care, for example blood sugar levels, without them having to visit the practice.

For simple requests such as these, email could be the answer. You need to be aware that:

- email—just like other messages—can go astray or be read by the wrong person
- you might not see the message straight away
- the message may be altered or deleted before you see it
- emails may be read by other practice staff, especially if you are away
- emails sent to your patients may be read by others who have access to their computer.

If you think email is a viable option for you and your practice, you need to decide whether or not you will charge for this service. At present there is no Medicare item number to cover this cost. You need to make sure your patients understand this if you intend to charge them.

REMEMBER!

Good communication is essential in the doctor–patient relationship. Email can supplement that relationship, but you are under no obligation to offer this service.

WHAT ARE THE RULES FOR USING EMAIL?

You and your patients will need to agree on the rules for using email, including how soon they can expect a reply.

It is a good idea to ask them to sign a form as part of that agreement and add it to their record. An example of such a form is shown in Figure 1.1. This is particularly important if you use email frequently with a number of patients. Not having an agreement in writing is likely to lead to misunderstanding at some stage.

FIGURE 1.1 EXAMPLE OF AN EMAIL AUTHORISATION FORM

(Practice name)

(Practice address line 1)

(Practice address line 2)

(Practice address line 3)

I acknowledge that Dr (First name) (Surname) and I have discussed the benefits and risks of using email to communicate with each other.

I understand my GP's practice will take all reasonable steps to keep my health information secure and private.

I agree only to use email for non-urgent matters, or to let the practice know if I move practices or change my email address.

My current email address is (please print):

Full name (please print):

Signed:

General practitioner's name (please print):

Signed: Date   /   / 20

Points to consider:
- If you receive an email from a patient who has not signed a form, ask them to make an appointment to discuss the matter.
- Check your email messages daily, as you would for phone messages or incoming test results.

- Respond to emails within the agreed timeframe. Aim for the same time in which you would return a phone call. Two working days is reasonable.
- Do not use email for bad news or sensitive matters.
- Give simple, clear responses.

HOW SAFE IS EMAIL?

Email can be a useful tool to deal with simple requests. But is it safe? And will it alter the risk of being sued?

You cannot guarantee the confidentiality of email, so you must take care when using it to communicate with patients. For example, non-authorised people might have access to your computer, or you might accidentally forward on the email to the wrong person. Viruses can also forward on your email without you knowing it. While the risk of email getting into the wrong hands might appear to be low, it does seem higher than for paper documents and, obviously, the precautions are different.

WHAT CAN I DO TO PROTECT INFORMATION AND MYSELF?

The following are some steps you can take to protect information and yourself:
- Set up password protection on all computers that receive emails from patients.
- Create email accounts that are specific to your general practice so that patient emails are not downloaded to your home computer.
- Make sure backups of your system include your email correspondence.
- Keep copies of all emails you send and receive. You can save all emails in separate folders for each patient, cut and paste them into the electronic medical record, or print and attach them to your paper record.
- Include a standard footer on all your emails—Figure 1.2 provides a good example.

HOW CAN I MAKE EMAIL WORK FOR MY PATIENTS AND ME?

You've made the decision to communicate with your patients by email. The following recommendations will help you make the most of this useful tool.

Do:
- update your policies and procedures manual to include a section on use of email (these policies should cover most of the matters referred to below)
- provide an information sheet on how you use email in your practice
- add all emails to the patient record—the patient should also keep a copy

FIGURE 1.2 EXAMPLE OF AN EMAIL FOOTER

Dr (First name) (Surname) MBBS FRACGP
Hillsdale General Practice
123 Ferny Crescent
Hillsdale Qld 4321

Email firstname.surname@hillsdalegp.com.au
Phone 02 1234 5678
Fax 02 1234 5688
Out of hours 02 1234 6666

....

Please do not use email for urgent matters; telephone either the practice or the emergency services.

This email, including any attachments, is confidential and for the sole use of the intended recipient(s). This confidentiality is not waived or lost if you receive it and you are not the intended recipient(s).

If you are not the intended recipient(s), you are asked to immediately notify the sender by telephone or by return email. You should also delete this email and destroy any hard copies produced.

- treat emails as official correspondence
- check for accuracy and appropriateness of language before sending
- include the full text of any previous emails with your reply to ensure you and the patient both know what you are referring to
- follow up with the patient to clarify details
- ask the patient to put their full name in the body of the email
- ask the patient to state the category or nature of the transaction in the subject line of the message so that it can be filtered (e.g. 'billing question')
- ask the patient to notify the practice if they change their email address or no longer wish to receive messages by email
- use the 'read receipt' and 'automatic reply' functions of your email system, and request that your patients do the same
- establish a system for checking the inboxes of absent staff, or set the system to forward their incoming messages automatically. Make sure you obtain their consent.

Don't:

- use email for anything urgent
- put anything in an email you wouldn't want added to the patient record
- initiate contact via email, except to provide a reminder
- respond to any email address other than the one agreed on. Contact the patient to inform them you need authorisation to respond to their enquiry at the new email address
- respond to emails from patients who are not registered with your practice.

REMEMBER!

The same rules apply to emails as to any other information stored in the practice. You need to take steps to make sure emails stay private and secure.

Case study **1.3**

It has been 2 weeks since you last saw Melanie. You receive an email from her in which she requests a prescription for temazepam, which her previous clinic had given her.

1 How do you handle this request?

2 What follow-up do you provide for Melanie, and what processes do you put in place for future email requests by her?

Computers, general practice and the law

WHAT IS MEANT BY 'THE LAW'?

'The law' comes from two sources:

- case law—also known as common law. These are the legal principles that have developed over time through the decisions of judges. Examples include the duty to exercise reasonable care in clinical service delivery, as required by the common law of negligence and the common law obligation of doctor–patient confidentiality.
- statute law—these are the legal obligations imposed by an Act of Parliament. Examples are legislation relating to privacy, drug prescription and access to records.

Together, these spell out what can, must and should be done to discharge legal obligations relevant to computing practices.

DO LEGAL OBLIGATIONS FOR COMPUTING DIFFER FROM OTHER GENERAL PRACTICE LEGAL OBLIGATIONS?

The law recognises that as a GP you occupy a special and important position of trust and confidentiality. This confers great powers but also involves significant responsibilities.

Your legal obligations in relation to privacy and confidentiality are the same, regardless of whether you use paper or a computer. Also, computers do not alter what patients can rightfully expect from you as their treating doctor.

Regardless of the setting in which services are being delivered, good communication, good documentation, good policies and good monitoring of those policies are crucial in ensuring that you and your staff discharge your legal obligations.

The same general principles will always apply. For example:

- The legal limits on how you collect, use and disclose patient information are unchanged. You must meet your legal responsibilities under privacy legislation and under common law confidentiality.
- The law of negligence requires you to exercise reasonable care. You will also be legally responsible for the negligence of your employees, under the principle of vicarious responsibility. The law will expect you and your staff to exercise reasonable care to maximise the potential and minimise the risks of computing practices.
- Using a computerised system does not affect your obligation to communicate clearly and effectively with patients.

Eventually, when most GPs include computing as one of their basic skills, the law will require all practitioners and their staff to be skilled to a defined standard. If you have already embraced the technology, you are required to exercise reasonable care when using it to conduct your services.

Changes have been made to the law to accommodate the challenges presented by technology (e.g. the introduction of electronic commerce legislation). However, the legal standing of some emerging forms of clinical interaction, only made possible by information and communications technology, has not yet been tested.

REMEMBER!

The law generally imposes the same obligations on GPs in the electronic environment as it does in the traditional setting.

WHAT LEGAL ISSUES AND RISKS DO I NEED TO CONSIDER?

You will need to exercise the same level of care and caution in managing your practice and patients as has always been required.

Working in a computing environment may mean you and your staff will use new tools in new ways to collect and use information, and for diagnosis, treatment and care. It is important to reinforce certain commonsense precautions to ensure your computing practices comply with your legal and clinical obligations. The tips below will help in that regard.

HOW DO I KEEP WITHIN THE LAW?

Know what you are doing and know your limitations
- Make sure you and your relevant staff become proficient with the technology. You don't have to invest in all the 'bells and whistles', but if you choose to use it, you need to know how to use it safely.
- Ensure your use of the technology is appropriate for the situation.
- Promote an environment that encourages peer support and sharing of information management and information technology (IM/IT) knowledge and skills.

Understand risk management and insurance issues
- Tell insurers about your IM/IT practices, particularly if those practices involve you in more entrepreneurial or novel collaborative relationships such as cybermedicine, telehealth and service delivery via the Internet.
- Be particularly cautious and seek advice from insurers if IM/IT practices—whether deliberately or inadvertently—may involve your clinic in the provision of medical services outside the jurisdiction for which it is registered, for example online consultations ('e-consultations').

Creating and retaining health records
- Ensure that all clinical records—whether in hard copy or electronic—are created contemporaneously (made at the time of the relevant event) and are comprehensive.
- Electronically generated data generally has the same legal standing as paper records. It can be your best medicolegal ally or your worst enemy, depending on how you use it.

REMEMBER!

Attention to the basic principles of good computer usage is in everyone's best interests.

Thinking about all the information in this chapter, what steps do you and your practice colleagues need to take to ensure the following?

- Administrative staff are clear about their access rights to patient clinical information.
- Patients know how you collect, store and use electronic information in your practice.
- You know how to deal with email from patients, including what to do if a request is made to a doctor who is away on leave.
- Patients know how you use email in your practice.
- Administrative staff know how to handle email requests addressed to the practice rather than an individual doctor.

If you have not already done so, you should conduct a practice meeting to discuss the above issues. You should also develop policies on the use of email for staff and for patients. The latter could be in the form of a handout or leaflet.

Summary

This chapter reviewed the relatively recent computerisation of general practice, and the fact that many GPs are still learning how to make the best use of computers. The electronic era has led to the development of a new concept in clinical practice: the patient–doctor–computer relationship. There are several areas in which this relationship is important.

The first of these areas is in the ability of the doctor to maintain rapport with the patient and keep them the focus of the consultation. While this might seem obvious, it will mean that you will benefit by improving your keyboard skills, improving your knowledge of the computer programs you use and developing new skills in getting patients involved in their own health records.

The second concerns patient privacy, which requires some additional precautions when clinical records are held in computers. You should understand your legal obligations in an electronic environment, although good communication remains the best means of maintaining a trusting relationship with your patients.

A third area to consider is an emerging new method of communication between practices and patients—email. It is possible to introduce your patients to email contact with the practice in specific and contained ways: checking appointments, providing basic information and advising about practice procedures. It is important to document your agreement with patients who want to use email.

The introduction of the computer into clinical practice means that you will need to develop policies on how to create, store, use and secure electronic data. This includes access rights to electronic data and procedures for the transfer of data to other health care providers.

So far we have concentrated on the doctor–patient–computer triad. In the next chapter we will look at the practice systems that you need to put in place so that your computers can improve the efficiency of your practice and help provide your patients with a more comprehensive and systematic approach to clinical care.

Computers and practice management

Computers aren't magic devices—they do nothing by themselves. They have to be set up and maintained properly or they won't do their job. They can seem daunting, and the time required to plan and install a system and then get it going can seem hard to justify. However, once the system has been running for a while you and the practice will be more productive, better informed and better able to care for your patients.

CONTENTS

When you have completed this chapter, you will be able to:

- list the activities that computers can be used for in your practice
- identify the computer software and hardware requirements of your practice
- determine the installation and support requirements of your IT system
- document your practice IT system
- define the roles and responsibilities of practice staff in supporting your practice IT system
- develop a budget to install and maintain your practice IT system.

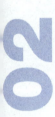

Introduction

What do you need to know about computers? How many do you need in your practice? What are they used for? What technical skills do you need at the practice, and what needs to be bought in?

This chapter describes some of the staff roles in installing and maintaining a computer system, and discusses the administrative functions of computers—the so-called 'front desk' functions such as billing, making appointments and establishing a patient database.

The chapter also looks at how your practice can connect to the Internet and communicate with other health care providers and organisations, including the government.

Clinical computing needs a system in which it can operate; this chapter will help you understand that system.

Note that mention of particular software packages is not meant as an endorsement of any one product over another—these are simply used as examples.

Computers in the practice—an overview

You can use a computer by itself or in conjunction with other computers as part of a network. The effort involved in setting up a network can be justified by its many advantages.

A computer can perform an array of tasks, in most cases simultaneously. Some tasks are inherent in the computer and its operating system, but most have to be set up and this often involves extra expenses, such as for software.

Computers come with their own jargon. The glossary of computer terminology at the end of the book will help you become familiar with this. You will also find some online reference sites, such as **www.webopedia.com**, which are useful to understanding the language of computers.

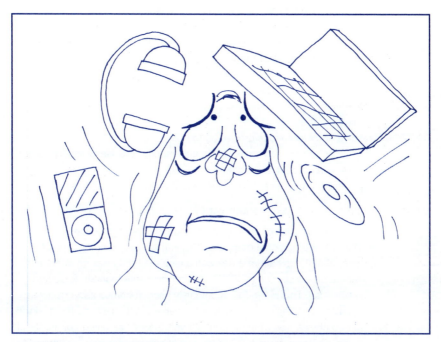

It's not easy being at the cutting edge of technology

WHAT CAN COMPUTERS DO IN THE PRACTICE?

Computers can save time, prevent mistakes and ensure that tasks are done in a consistent manner. However, some applications have little immediate value or practical use.

It is best to introduce just one or two applications when you first computerise, but it is important to allow for future applications in your planning. Make sure you have sufficient hardware and choose your software with your future needs in mind.

In a general practice, computers can allow you to:
- run specific software for clinical, practice management and accounting purposes
- create documents
- access the Internet

- store files (such as documents, images and data)
- print documents and images
- send and receive emails
- access reports from pathology providers and specialists
- share case notes and documents with other professionals
- access online groups
- access government financial claiming services
- further your studies
- access data (such as patient records) remotely
- send faxes (from and to the computer).
     Other possible uses include:
- specialised communications such as videoconferencing or Internet telephony
- teleconsulting
- voice entry (note taking or voice to text)
- voice output (text to speech), such as reading articles or reports to you while you do something else
- potential future uses, such as remote monitoring of patients.

WHAT DO I NEED TO KNOW ABOUT HARDWARE?

Three primary types of computer are used in general practice.
- The desktop personal computer (PC) is the most common type of computer. It consists of a box containing the hard drive, memory and central processing unit (CPU or 'brain'); separate monitor; keyboard and mouse. This is the PC traditionally used in homes and businesses.
- The notebook PC, or laptop, has the same functionality as the desktop, but combines everything in a single unit. As well as being adaptable to mains power, notebook PCs are usually battery-powered for portability.
- The 'thin client' is a relatively 'dumb' workstation, or older PC, connected to a server that provides the processing power. The PC in this case refers mainly to a screen, keyboard and mouse, with only a modest computer 'brain' of its own.

Computers in a practice can be stand-alone or networked. Networks offer a number of advantages:
- Many of the clinical and practice management systems will now only run from a server-based system.
- Your practice can share broadband Internet access and distribute it via the network.
- A networked system makes it much easier to provide basic, essential services such as backup and security.
- Versatility is enhanced—you can access information from any PC in the practice, or from a remote location.
- Different levels of access can be assigned to different users.

A local area network (LAN) traditionally connects various devices together by wiring, but wireless connections are increasingly being used for some or even all devices. You will almost certainly need to pay for professional IT assistance to set up a network in your practice.

WHAT IS WIRELESS NETWORKING?

Wireless networking uses radio signals to connect devices together. It has the following characteristics:
- It is inherently insecure, as others may be able to intercept the data.
- The range is typically 10 to 50 metres, although this can extend to kilometres.
- Other devices that use the same radio frequency (e.g. cordless phones) can cause intermittent access.
- A benefit is that it makes it easy to move a notebook computer between two or more locations, yet have network and Internet access without connecting a cable.

REMEMBER!
Understand the risks of wireless networking before you install it.

WHAT SOFTWARE DO I NEED?

Your software needs will depend on how far and how fast you want to go in computerising your practice. It is essential to have:
- a server operating system
- a workstation operating system.
  Additional options include:
- clinical packages
- a practice management package
- accounting software
- an office package for word processing and spreadsheets
- security utilities, such as antivirus and firewall (see Chapter 5 for more detail)
- any other software of choice.

Some functions, such as backing up, may be built into software or need to be bought as a stand-alone package.

Eventually you will replace or upgrade software with newer versions. You can receive service packs and bug fixes to maintain the software, but after about 3 years you will most likely need either a total replacement or upgrade.

DO I HAVE TO PAY FOR EACH PERSON TO USE THE SOFTWARE?

Some software—known as 'open source'—is available free of charge. Other software is proprietary and can only be used under licence.

In some cases the licence fee is payable once only, but in many cases payment of an annual fee is required, especially if you want to receive the latest software updates. This is especially so in the case of proprietary antivirus programs. These function effectively only if they are updated frequently (preferably daily) to ensure filtering of the latest viruses.

Make sure you know what you're paying for. You can either pay for each person who will use the software, or pay for a maximum number of concurrent users. The latter method is usually cheaper, especially if it allows you to load the software onto spare computers and notebooks for times when regular computers are out of service. Regardless of which you start with, you should be able to add new licences with little more than a phone call and a credit card.

Installing and maintaining the computers

02

A practice staff member can install and maintain your computer system, provided they have the expertise or are willing to learn. The more usual method is to hire someone to set up the computers and then, over time, learn to do more of the ongoing tasks yourself. The practice manager usually looks after the computer installation, using external help as necessary, but the responsibility could be taken by anyone.

WHAT IS THE BEST METHOD FOR SETTING UP MY COMPUTER SYSTEM?

Consult your colleagues and perhaps your local division before choosing one of the following methods. This will help you to avoid the most common mistakes.

- Find an external supplier or contractor who can set up some or all of the system. You may also contract them to maintain the system. This could be the local computer shop or a specialist recommended or even provided by the vendor of your practice software.
- Contract someone to supply, install and maintain the entire system for a fixed fee (e.g. $X per user per month for all requirements, including software). The advantage of this method is that all you have to do is learn to use the system.
- For the set-up phase, hire someone who has done similar jobs before, such as a practice manager or IT manager from another practice.
- Consider sharing the cost of hiring someone across a few practices.
- Do everything you can within the practice.

Increasingly, group practices have bitten the bullet and decided that coming to an arrangement with an experienced IT service is the best option. There will probably be a regular 'maintenance' fee, plus an additional call-out fee to fix problems or provide extra services.

The cost of the computer system has become just another business expense. However, some of the money can be recouped either by direct government payments (e.g. under the Practice Incentives Program run by the Australian Government), or by additional medical services which occur as a result of computer functions such as recall systems.

REMEMBER!

Keep track of your costs. Your computer, just like any other operating expense, is tax deductible. Investigate government financial incentives.

PRACTICAL EXERCISE

Make a list of what your practice IT requirements are for both hardware and software. What do you currently use? What tasks would you like to be able to do with your computer system? If you don't know, who in your practice does? Can you compile a list between the two of you? Do a tour of your practice and see what you have.

WHAT DOCUMENTATION DO I NEED?

No matter who sets up or maintains the system, it is essential to document everything, and to keep this log up-to-date. Personnel inevitably change and suppliers go out of business; you can't be expected to remember every important fact.

Some people maintain their system log as paper only. If you maintain it electronically, always have a full printout (if the system is down you won't be able to read the electronic version).

Keep the following information as a minimum:
- written and diagrammatic descriptions of the system and its purpose
- list of all hardware
- list of contacts of the various suppliers and maintainers of hardware, software and services (you should never be in the position of not knowing how to contact any person who may be needed)

- list of all software, including:
  - the number of licences
  - how the software is licensed
  - licence registration number
  - expiry date
- standard operating procedures, such as who is responsible for particular tasks and when these tasks should be done
- log of all system problems and how they were fixed (which may be useful in the future)
- log of all system modifications, who performed them, and a statement that the system was checked afterwards to ensure that both the new and existing system work
- list of jobs to be done (mandatory and wish list)
- log of all resources such as training materials and contacts.

The GPCG has a template for a log book. You can find it with other components of the GPCG computer security guidelines at **www.gpcg.org.au**

WHO IS RESPONSIBLE?

Someone in the practice should be responsible for the day-to-day maintenance of the system. Usually, the practice manager or senior receptionist takes on this role. You could do this yourself or hire someone specifically for the job, or share the position across two or more practices or locations.

Whoever looks after the system, you will need to make some decisions on:
- who enters data
- who has access to patient or financial information
- who is responsible for purchases and upgrades
- who is responsible for backing-up data.

All staff should be able to do some of the data entry. Everyone should have password access to systems they are authorised to read or modify. Some people will have specific jobs and some people will be authorised to assist. Some systems, such as the clinical software, will probably be limited to medical staff, including practice nurses.

You will decide who has access to what information. By default, most software will require someone (i.e. your system manager) to assign access to each module, rather than deny it.

DO I STILL NEED TO KEEP PAPER RECORDS?

The legal standing is not entirely clear regarding the length of time you should keep paper or electronic records. Here are some rules of thumb:
- the value of a record is dependent on its physical safety. Always keep a backup copy in a different location

- you don't need to print a document that has been generated electronically simply for the sake of having a copy on paper
- you can scan a paper document and store it as an electronic image or convert it to text by optical character recognition (OCR) software. However, keep in mind that scanned documents may be problematic in a court of law (see Chapter 1 for a discussion about the legal aspects of this topic)
- if a document originates in hard copy format then you should probably keep it in that format for the legally required period.

When setting up a new system, you will need to decide what to do with your paper health records. Most practices find that running two systems—paper and electronic—for some time is the best solution. You decide on a particular date when new records are entered electronically, but you keep the paper records on hand. It might be feasible to scan all of your previous records into an electronic form, but larger practices find this a rather overwhelming task. It seems easier to write electronic summaries of paper records as patients come to the practice. The problem with this approach is that you could be running the two systems together for some years, which is frustrating.

Discuss the options with your staff and decide which method is most efficient and cost effective in your circumstances.

> **REMEMBER!**
> Electronic records are admissible in court, but scanned images are less reliable as they can be altered. Play it safe and keep the original.

HOW DO I KNOW MY DATA IS SECURE?

There are two essential aspects of using computers in your practice: backup (against data being lost or corrupted) and security (against data falling into the wrong hands). The particular characteristics of electronic records over paper records are that:
- hardware and software can fail, leading to a loss of computer data— hence the need to create a backup
- electronic records can be accessed remotely by unauthorised people— hence the need to put in place a number of computer security measures.

Chapter 5 goes into computer security in considerable detail, so there is no need to explain much at this point. However, you need to make decisions about computer security when setting up your system; you cannot leave this till later.

HOW DO I GET COMPUTER TECHNICAL SUPPORT WHEN I NEED IT?

The best person or organisation to support the system will most likely be the one who supplied and installed it.

You could employ a technical support person who is trained in your clinical and practice management software, and who may even support other practices in the area. Alternatively, someone in the practice could take on some of the support role. In this case it is important to have a procedure for handling a problem if it can't be solved within the office. Always have one person whose responsibility it is to contact outside help services.

You should also have a system in place for continuing the business when all or part of the system is down. This should include a straightforward method of incorporating any manual records made during this period into the system once it is restored (see Chapter 5).

REMEMBER!

It is important to log all system problems and their resolution.

HOW MUCH WILL IT COST TO COMPUTERISE?

There is no easy way to put a price on computerisation. You can talk to other practices or your division of general practice to get some costing guidelines, but if you are very new to computer technology, consider purchasing your computers as a package that includes service-level guarantees.

The cost of an installation includes many more components than you might first imagine. Table 2.1 lists some examples.

> **REMEMBER!**
>
> Weigh up the costs and advantages of each computer equipment purchase. Consider the ongoing costs. For example, you may pay less for an inkjet printer than a laser printer—but will replacement ink cartridges result in a greater cost in the long run?

TABLE 2.1 TYPICAL COSTS OF INFORMATION TECHNOLOGY (IN AUSTRALIAN DOLLARS)

Item	Cost
HARDWARE	
• server	• $1000–5000
• workstation	• $800–2000
• LCD monitor	• $300–1500
• notebook PC	• $900–5000
• printer	• $60–6000
• backup system	• $200–5000
• networking infrastructure	• This can be as basic as a network cable running along the floor for $100, to a professional rewiring job costing many thousands of dollars
• Internet gateway and firewall box	• $150–2000
• wireless networking access point	• $150–400
• scanner	• $100–1000
• web camera	• $40–2000
• uninterruptible power supply (UPS)	• $200–5000
SOFTWARE	
• office programs (such as Microsoft Office)	• $500–1200 per user
• clinical package	• $200–1000 per user per year
• practice management package	• $200–1000 per user per year
• accounting package	• $200–1000 per user per year
TRAINING (including time to learn an application)	Cost will vary enormously between practices, depending on existing knowledge. The bulk of the cost is your time. Trainers may charge between $30 and $200 per hour or more
TECHNICAL SUPPORT	$40–150 per hour
CONSUMABLES	
• inkjet print (black)	• 5–15¢ per A4 page
• inkjet print (colour)	• 25¢ to $6 per A4 page
• laser print (black)	• 2–10¢ per A4 page
• electricity	• Less than $1 per person per day (more for equipment left on overnight)
• CD or DVD for backup storage	• 20¢ to $4 each
INTERNET ACCESS	Typical broadband access costs between $30 and $300 per month

Practice management software

Clinical programs help with consultations but practice management software keeps your business healthy. These programs keep track of billing, claiming, electronic lodgements and debts, and hence improve income and cash flow.

WHICH IS THE BEST SOFTWARE PACKAGE?

The practice management system should be compatible with your preferred database, operating systems and other technologies. Can the program link with your clinical software? This saves time and avoids the unnecessary double entry of patient details by GPs and staff. Many packages are now fully integrated, so the issue of program linkage is becoming less of a problem.

When choosing software, you should consider:
- cost—remember to plan for installation, training and upgrades
- expected growth of the practice—more GPs means additional software licences which may have to support multisite operations
- time involved in maintaining and backing-up data
- level of technical support provided by the software vendor.

If you are moving from an all-manual system, will the transition be smooth? Can you do it as you go or will you have to spend long hours working before it is ready for the first use? Gather some first-hand opinions of what these programs are like to use from other GPs and practice managers.

Practice management programs typically provide:
- appointments
- waiting room management
- 'private' and 'bulk' billing (the latter means billing the government rather than the patient)
- electronic claiming (i.e. the ability to electronically send a batch of bulk-billed service invoices to the government), which in Australia is called Medicare's Online Claiming system
- electronic lodgements and reporting features.

Investigate those features that are important to you and your practice.

WHAT SHOULD I LOOK FOR IN A DATABASE?

Your database is the core of your practice management system. You need a robust database that will protect your data from corruption. It should:
- be able to grow with your practice (and handle an ever-increasing volume of information)

- include useful utilities for backup, verification and integrity checking
- be able to export the information to other databases.

Different products rely on different kinds of databases, which in turn may require certain operating systems and hardware. Depending on the database required for your choice of practice management software, you may need additional licensing.

HOW DO I ENTER DATA?

Patient registration must be convenient, with enough fields to allow you to record all relevant details and make use of this information in searching or sorting.

Some systems can import patient data from other sources, such as Medicare (listing patients your practice has claimed for) or pathology providers (patients you have sent for tests).

You will need to enter many patient details by hand (such as notes), so look for an easy interface with plenty of helpful fields (not just names and addresses), and areas for adding special notes or details (e.g. a workers compensation claim reference number). Other features to consider are intuitive data entry, calculators and look-up tables.

Once the database is set up, you should be able to find any information you want, quickly and easily. You should be able to search for information by text, using the same sorts of techniques you use in Internet searches. You should also be able to create structured queries and views that you can save for use on future occasions.

You should be able to export data and use it for other purposes, such as creating mailing lists for a newsletter or transferring a patient's records to another surgery.

HOW DO I KEEP TRACK OF APPOINTMENTS?

The database's appointments facility should be able to specify GPs, nurses, rooms and any special equipment required. You should be able to define intervals between appointments, book a long consultation and block out time for a meeting.

A waiting room module allows front desk staff to keep track of who has turned up and gives you a chance to check how long your next patient has been waiting before asking them in. The practice management software should link to the patient record so that you can quickly call it up as the patient comes in to the consulting room.

HOW WILL SOFTWARE HELP WITH BILLING?

Your practice management software will improve the billing process. It should be flexible enough to:
- cope with various billing situations and parties (e.g. Medicare, Department of Veterans' Affairs, insurance companies)

- add other GPs or locums to stationery (computer-generated letterheads and forms save costs)
- streamline billing and claiming to improve cash flow and income
- help you ensure patients have been correctly billed and identify parties who have not paid
- prompt you about your entitlements or about small amounts owed from different sources (e.g. the Australian Childhood Immunisation Register). Electronic lodging makes it easier to report an immunisation and be credited.

Such management is essential for private billing, but it can also help make bulk billing a more reliable income stream through prompt lodgement with the government (e.g. Medicare Australia).

CAN I GENERATE FINANCIAL REPORTS?

You will be able to generate a range of reports about billing, income and demographics for the practice (such as the percentage of patients with a certain status) or for individual doctors. You will be able to check a day sheet, confirm which patients you've seen and if they've been correctly billed, or check on that day's earnings. Reports allow you to print reminders for overdue accounts.

PRACTICAL EXERCISE

Do you know what you want from your practice management program? What information has to be on a patient invoice and receipt? What sort of financial reports do you wish to generate? Does this program need to integrate with an accounting package? What are the differences in the functionalities of appointment systems of one program compared with another? Do you want to make appointments from your own desktop, or pass that responsibility to your receptionist?

Follow your practice management program's functions from the time a patient arrives at the front desk, through the consultation and when they return to the front desk before leaving. At the very least, see how the appointment and billing systems work.

Electronic links

WHY DO I NEED THE INTERNET?

A broadband Internet connection is increasingly seen as essential for operating a medical practice. With an Internet connection you will be able to:

- access reference and educational information for you and your patients to read
- communicate with patients via your practice website
- perform specialised real-time communications such as videoconferencing and Internet telephone calls
- engage in teleconsulting
- access Medicare's Online Claiming to lodge medical service claims
- do online banking.

HOW DO I CONNECT TO THE INTERNET?

Most general practices are able to connect via asymmetrical digital subscriber line (ADSL). Normally you need to be within 4 kilometres of a telephone exchange that is equipped for ADSL. You also need the correct type and quality of phone line.

Virtually all practices are able to connect to broadband by some method, although some rural practices may find it more difficult.

There are alternatives to ADSL. Many areas, especially metropolitan ones, will have cable Internet available. This uses a fibre-optic cable which is also used to distribute television programs. Even if you are completely isolated and without a phone line, you should be able to access the Internet via a satellite connection provided you have clear access to the sky. There can be disadvantages in using satellite, such as an extra delay in voice and video conferencing (about half a second). Various other types of wireless Internet services exist, including community-based distribution systems that you may be able to access (or create).

The Australian Government has provided subsidised Internet connections to GPs under its 'Broadband for Health' scheme (go to **www.health.gov.au** and enter 'broadband for health' into the site's search engine). Although the financial incentives are unlikely to continue for much longer, the government has tried to ensure that Internet service providers deliver 'business grade' Internet connections to general practice, that is, connections with basic standards and securities guaranteed.

WHAT DO I NEED TO SEND EMAILS?

You will need an Internet connection and the appropriate software. All email systems interconnect automatically—messages created in one software package will always be compatible with those connected to another. The basic email program in Windows is Outlook Express. A number of other email systems offer more features—for example, Outlook, which is part of Microsoft Office, or free software packages such as Mozilla's Thunderbird.

With a little practice, you can teach yourself to become quite proficient at using email. Spending a little time reading the Help section of the particular program you are using will teach you all you need to know. Although you will have to be careful how you use this handy tool with patients, you will find many other uses for it. Some practices use email as an internal communication device. For example, 'front desk' staff can place non-urgent prescription requests on email rather than the 'sticky notes' which might not be kept confidential. Chapter 1 deals with some of the practical and ethical issues in communicating with patients by email.

Chapter 5 introduces the subject of email encryption which is a method of 'scrambling' the message so that only the intended recipient can read it. This helps to keep electronic communication private and secure.

WHAT IS 'INTEROPERABILITY' AND HOW WILL IT AFFECT ELECTRONIC COMMUNICATION IN THE FUTURE?

Electronic communication is much more than you being able to access the Internet or send and receive emails. It is also more than being able to download pathology results. In the hopefully not too distant future, you will be part of an electronic health network in which you can easily exchange patient clinical data with hospitals, medical specialists, allied health professionals and others. Obviously, this will have to occur within agreed privacy guidelines.

What has to happen in order to be electronically connected? People sometimes say that computers have to be able to 'talk' to each other. Others with a penchant for tongue twisters call it 'interoperability' (say that three times quickly).

Interoperability is quite a complex process. It can be defined as the ability to transfer and use information in a uniform and efficient manner across multiple organisations and computer systems. It is easiest to understand what this means by breaking it down into its component parts: technical, semantic and business process interoperability.

• Technical interoperability. In order for data to be able to move from one system to another, there have to be agreed *standards* on how electronic data is communicated, transported, stored and represented. Let's illustrate this by two brief examples:
  – HL7 is a clinical messaging standard which can be used to send pathology data from a laboratory to a clinician's computer. It defines the electronic record and how the data should appear within it. HL7 is like a 'wrapper' for a pathology result so that it can be transported and then incorporated into the electronic medical record.
  – Public key infrastructure (PKI) is a data security standard which provides a means to encrypt and decrypt data, and authenticates who sent and who received it.

For two computer systems to be technically interoperable via a network, there has to be agreement on the use of common 'standards'.

- Semantic interoperability. Words have to have consistent meaning, especially when they are transferred from one system to another. For example, laboratories might use either the term 'glycated haemoglobin' or 'glycosylated haemoglobin'. This lack of consistency in terminology makes it difficult for you to search electronically which of your patients with diabetes have had this test, or what the mean value is. Agreement on using defined terms is important in the following areas:
  - clinical codes for diagnostic categories (examples of coding systems are SNOMED-CT and ICD-10)
  - codes for pathology tests and medication
  - a core dataset of words (vocabulary) to describe what takes place in a clinical encounter.
- Business process interoperability. Human beings—not computers—have to reach an understanding on how to use the network. This involves putting in place systems to ensure:
  - clear decision making and accountability on such matters as the choice of technical standards
  - training programs for users of the system
  - a legal framework within which users operate
  - a 'directory' of members of the network which is kept up-to-date.

As you can see, getting computers to 'talk to each other' involves a lot of separate things. Getting computers to understand the message is even harder! Getting a group of people to agree on all of these has historically been a very hard task. For example, much debate has taken place within Australia on which are the best technical standards to use in e-health. As people become frustrated with the lack of progress, there are calls for the government to mandate the use of standards—any standards—just so that something gets done. But so far this has not happened.

What has happened is that individual companies have come up with their own solutions. For example, pathology laboratories can use a service company to transfer pathology data to GPs who wish to receive results electronically. All the GPs need to do is allow the company to install company-specific software on their computers. This is an example of a 'point-to-point' solution. It works very well, but how many individual solutions are practical? What we really want is for the whole system to be 'interoperable'!

Is this important for general practice? Yes it is, because we are edging our way towards an electronic health record that can be shared by a number of health care providers—with patient consent—giving GPs better information during a consultation.

Have you considered the following about Internet connections to your practice?

1 What type of Internet connection can you get in your area, and why does this matter?
2 Are there any particular issues you should know about if your Internet connection is from a computer that is a part of a local area network (LAN)?
3 Can you access your computer system remotely (e.g. when on house calls or at home)?

Make some enquires with colleagues about their Internet connections, including remote access. What would work best for your practice?

Summary

You should now have a better understanding of your practice's hardware and software requirements. This chapter should also have helped you appreciate that, as well as technical knowledge, you need some understanding of how the implementation and integration of computerisation will work with support from various members of staff—doctors, administrative staff and, when required, IT technical support.

Computers and clinical care

This chapter looks at key issues in the use of computers in clinical care. It is about using the computer on your desk to improve the care of patients.

CONTENTS

(cont. overleaf)

LEARNING OBJECTIVES

When you have completed this chapter, you will be able to:

- appreciate the advantages of electronic health records over paper-based ones
- define the roles and responsibilities of practice staff to support data entry and the integrity of computer records
- plan a timetable for the implementation of electronic health records in your practice
- identify the training needs and implement a training program, so practice staff can confidently and competently perform their data entry tasks
- identify the procedures in transferring relevant health data from paper files to the electronic record
- define the relevant data to be entered in each category of the electronic health summary
- understand the importance of coding health information
- list the advantages and disadvantages of drug allergy and interaction warnings
- demonstrate the use of the electronic health record in the consultation, ensuring the accuracy of a range of clinical data
- demonstrate the use of the computer for
  - creating and storing health summaries
  - prescribing
  - handling patient investigations
  - using templates
  - implementing recalls and reminders
  - searching the patient database
  - using decision-support tools that are part of the clinical software.

Introduction

Some GPs use clinical software just to write prescriptions; others have more advanced computer skills. You need to decide what you want from your computer. This chapter explains how you can use more of these tools to gain maximum benefit from your computer as your knowledge and confidence increases.

We begin with some of the basics, such as how to add patients to the database and how to transfer records from a paper-based system to an electronic one. We then describe various aspects of clinical software—the health summary, the prescribing functions, past history, allergy warnings and so on. Some of the topics require not only computer skills, but an understanding of how such a system works at a practice level. For example, how do you ensure that patients with abnormal test results are notified?

The chapter explains the particular benefits of computers in chronic disease management and using a recall and reminder system. These demonstrate the advantages of computers over paper records.

In this chapter we will review the major requirements of moving from paper records to computer records. We will consider how computers can alter and improve clinical practice. There are several software packages available for general practice and the principles that are outlined in this chapter apply to all of them.

The computer record

Unlike the paper record, the computer can assist with a range of functions in the background, during the consultation. The computer can help with many clinical tasks—prescribing is the classic example, with background checking of allergies, drug and disease interactions.

HOW DO I ADD NEW PATIENT RECORDS?

Enter the data for new patients at the front desk and 'link' it to the medical record from the practice management software. This ensures that the medical record is ready when the patient arrives in your consulting room. You don't need separate software for medical records and accounting. The duplication of data entry is time consuming and prone to error.

Practice staff should be responsible for all the simple demographic data and other information that supports the billing systems, but,

generally, unless they have had specific training, your receptionist should not enter medical record data because:
- the information is confidential and personal
- they may not sufficiently understand the medical terminology
- any errors in data entry become your responsibility as the practitioner.

Practice nurses can enter a large part of the initial medical record data. They can interview new patients to set up the recall and prevention process of the computer system. For patients with chronic disease or significant health risk factors this would establish a sound foundation and process for regular, evidence-based monitoring.

Encourage your nursing staff to use the electronic record, and ensure they receive the same degree of training as the medical practitioners. Most software packages offer excellent tools in the area of health promotion, prevention and public health, which can facilitate the role of practice nurses. Use this to enhance your overall service and improve overall patient care.

HOW DO I TRANSFER OLD MEDICAL RECORDS?

Old records can be either paper-based or electronic files.

Transferring paper records

The quality of paper records can vary widely. Where the record is not current or is poor, it is best to check all details with the patient.

If electronic scanning is available, scan any key paper records. Otherwise, you could record a short summary in the electronic record under the relevant chronic health problem.

Transferring electronic records

The key issue here will be the compatibility of old and new electronic records. Import the old record into the new one if you are able. Check the old data for accuracy with your patient at their next visit, especially the health summary, which the patient could check as a printed copy.

Where your new and old software are incompatible, you can often import the information as a straight text file but this is of limited value. If you don't know whether the old and new software are compatible, then ignore the old data and start a new record, but include a summary of the old one by entering this manually.

Scanning

Scanning a paper document allows you to store it as an electronic image or convert it to text. There are two methods of scanning: scanning as an image or picture of the document and optical character recognition (OCR). The benefits of scanning are that you can:
- store documents in the electronic record
- include images or photographs in the record

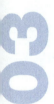

- search an OCR-converted document for words in the text and as part of a search of the entire medical record system.

  However, there are drawbacks:
- Electronic records are admissible in court, but as scanned images can be altered their legal status is diminished. You may therefore choose to keep some original documents for medicolegal reasons.
- Scanned images can take up a lot of disk space.
- Scanning can create confidentiality issues. The person scanning needs to check each page and read at least some of the material, and therefore should be someone authorised to access the information.
- The process is time consuming.

Health summary

The health summary is an overview of information held in the electronic medical record. The computer-based health summary:
- updates automatically when information is changed
- does not require the same maintenance process as the paper equivalent
- will be current and should be the entry point to any consultation.

REMEMBER!

Failure to check the health summary when reviewing the patient is likely to be considered poor practice. It would be difficult to defend an adverse outcome where this was not done.

You can choose what to include in the health summary and the order in which it is presented, or work with the default option.

WHAT SORT OF INFORMATION DO I INCLUDE IN THE HEALTH SUMMARY?

Demographic information
This covers the basic details about a patient: address, phone contact, email, date of birth, Medicare and private insurance details, entitlements and next of kin.

Identify and correct any errors or omissions in this information during the consultation
The computer retains the demographic information as part of the key patient master file. This is the base of any searches of reports on patients, including all the recall and screening reports and letters. Thus, decide what demographic information is important when choosing a computer software package. One particular advantage of the computer system is the automatic calculation and presentation of a patient's age.

Family and social history

Family and social history is generally in unstructured free text. It makes no functional contribution to managing your patient. It appears conveniently in the health summary and can be readily included in letter templates for referrals or other communication.

When you record an important family risk factor, you must move to a recall screen to apply the corresponding protocol to address that risk. You should record important family health risks as a separate ongoing health problem. Genetic or DNA information is likely to reside in this area and may replace traditional family history.

Commonly recorded social history information includes:

- immediate family structure
- sports, hobbies and interests
- education and work history
- key life events (e.g. migration).

Future software development will allow you to track information. For example, it will be helpful when programs automatically update the record when one family member is diagnosed with an illness that may affect others. Or you might be able to search for and generate a recall for any worker who has worked with an organisation that handles asbestos.

Measurements

The computer is ideal for recording and presenting measurements in a graphical form, especially percentile charts:

- Height is mostly recorded in centimetres.
- Weight is recorded in kilograms.
- Body mass index will be calculated from the last recorded height and weight. Some computer systems can graph this measurement. Many clinicians acknowledge that waist measurement or body fat measurement may be better indicators, but software packages vary in their ability to record this information.
- Blood pressure is recorded separately as systolic and diastolic. Some software will allow the separate recording of sitting, lying and standing

pressures. Generally, you can graph either diastolic or systolic blood pressure, but not necessarily both on the same graph.
- Respiratory function is available in the electronic record to varying degrees including:
  - simply recording lung function measurements
  - recording with normal values evident
  - recording data directly from common vitalograph machines
  - pre- and post-bronchodilator recording (generally available with comparison)
  - graphing of results.
- Most software can record blood glucose and HbA1C. You can also upload information from some glucometers. Some software allows quite sophisticated graphing of fasting and random blood glucose levels.
- Most software can record cholesterol and the other elements of the lipid profile. You may have to enter the data into the examination fields in the progress notes. Few packages have the facility to take the cholesterol information from results downloaded from the pathologist, although this is increasingly possible as test results are written in a standardised (i.e. HL7) format.

HOW DO I RECORD SMOKING, ALCOHOL AND OTHER DRUG USE?

Some features are not available in all software. Research the software package to see whether it has the tools you need.

Smoking

Key smoking information will appear on the health summary; however, it is more prominent when recorded as a health problem. Given the importance of smoking in disease prevention, it is important to flag the fact that a patient is a current smoker.
- Current habit is recorded in all medical record software. Record smoking as an active health problem, as this is not automatic.
- Smoking history can at least be recorded with a commencement date and the number of years the patient has smoked. You cannot generally record changes over time. At least one software package has the useful feature of recording all changes when they are entered in the progress notes.
- 'Readiness to quit' is a tool that provides a short questionnaire gauging and recording a patient's readiness to quit. This is a useful reminder when recording smoking history; use it to prompt the development of a quit plan.
- 'History of attempts to quit' records details of the last attempt and successful quit period.

You should be able to produce a list of smokers and generate a letter promoting information on quitting.

Alcohol

Alcohol use does not appear in the health summary produced by most software packages. Record it as an active health problem.

The key issue for clinical care is the quantity of alcohol being consumed. Few software packages manage this very well, but some now include a small alcohol questionnaire. This is useful, but it will be better when the average daily usage is calculated.

Other drug use

Currently available software doesn't record other drug use, including illicit drugs. You can record it in free text under the social history. One difficulty with illicit drug use is the issue of confidentiality. Some software allows you to flag illicit drug use as confidential. This means only the treating doctor can see the health problem on the summary list. Unless your patient has a significant health problem, the health summary generally doesn't record drug use.

Past medical history

Past medical history is an inconsistent feature across the various software packages. In some packages active, inactive, chronic and past health problems are recorded in past history. Other packages classify health problems as current or past, and allow you to move problems from past to current or vice versa.

HOW IMPORTANT IS IT TO CODE INFORMATION?

Coding is simple, and is essential for retrieving information later. It allows the computer to run complex background activities, such as:

- checking drug interactions against a patient's known health problems
- recalls for patients with chronic health problems
- research and auditing
- government health incentive programs (e.g. diabetes).

The computer will attempt to recognise each health problem as it is entered. Working out the quickest way to record common health problems does not take long as the actual coding happens in the background and in most systems this will not be obvious to the user.

WILL I BE ABLE TO RECORD INFORMATION RELEVANT TO A PAST PROBLEM?

Ideally, you should be able to record the following relevant information about a patient's problem:

- the title of the problem, with associated background coding
- the date it commenced

- whether it is active or inactive
- whether it should be included in the health summary
- whether it is confidential (this affects who can see the problem in the summary)
- the date it was resolved
- notes in the free text area.

You won't be able to record this in all software, so again, choose your software carefully according to your needs. If your practice deals with a great deal of chronic disease, then your software needs to have a sophisticated approach to health problems.

In particular, your software should easily set the date on which a health problem is resolved, and easily change health problems from active to inactive. Software should allow a space to record a free text note on each health problem.

Prescribing

HOW DO COMPUTERS AFFECT PRESCRIBING?

A major benefit of using computers to prescribe is increased safety for the patient and the doctor. Computer use can result in more appropriate prescriptions, a vital part of providing quality care.

Computers can provide notification of:
- allergies recorded to a drug or class of drugs
- possible drug interactions
- possible drug and disease interactions
- alternative treatments.

Computers can also provide drug prices, and much of the information found in the Pharmaceutical Benefits Schedule. However, the time required to read and consider the computer's warnings and advice may add to the duration and complexity of the consultation.

There are many other benefits of computer prescribing:
- It saves time.
- Prescriptions are more legible.
- You can access a current prescribing information database.
- You can use either trade or generic names.
- You can link a medication to a particular problem and generate a list of relevant medications.
- It provides an accurate, current medication list.
- Some software packages allow you to set up drug protocols for particular situations (e.g. prescribing several medications to travellers to a certain region).

- You can store particular instructions as well as the standard set available (e.g. specifying the use of a medication for a particular purpose for a short time).
  There are also limitations:
- You need to know how to record whether a prescription is a one-off (such as an antibiotic) or a continuing medication (such as an antihypertensive).
- It is easy to generate a prescription for a patient, but if you forget to change that patient's details in their electronic record, you may end up with a prescription in the incorrect name. Always check.
- It is easy to click on the wrong medication in a list of similar names.
- The warnings vary in reliability.
- Standard drug databases risk losing the old recipe prescriptions (particularly evident in dermatology in the past).

REMEMBER!

Always check any computer prescription before handing it to the patient. Make sure it's the intended medication, for the intended patient.

WHAT WARNINGS AND ADVICE CAN THE COMPUTER PROVIDE?

Allergy warnings

Allergy warnings—drug and non-drug—will only work if the allergy has been recorded in the system. Maintain normal clinical practice and always ask the patient before prescribing.

Drug allergies can be identified by generic name, trade name or group. Non-drug allergies are generally displayed as free text and will not be recorded as a health problem in the health summary, although the allergy will be listed in the allergies field.

Drug interaction warnings

You can set this interaction to different levels of sensitivity to exclude less relevant interactions. You can ignore or overrule a warning, but you will always see the warning first. You will not be able to deny being warned by the system in the event of an adverse outcome. Most warning systems provide sufficient detail to allow you to make a decision without seeking further reference.

This warning system is not reliable with respect to alternative medicines.

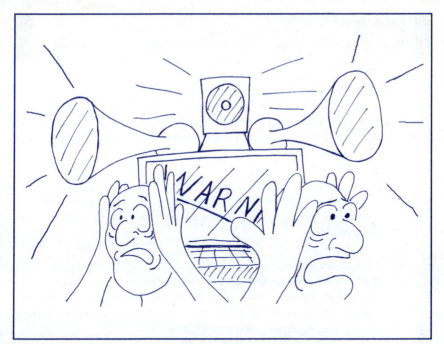

Make sure you don't overlook any warning messages

> **REMEMBER!**
>
> It is vital that you have an up-to-date medication list for each patient if the warning system is to operate effectively and safely.

Health problem and drug interaction warnings
This feature depends on how you code the health problem. For example, you may be warned about prescribing a beta blocker for a patient with asthma, but not for one with bronchitis or a variant of asthma.

No software packages should be wholly relied on as a warning system—they offer a limited, but still useful, back up.

General warnings: pregnancy and elite sport
The computer will generally warn you to check prescribed medication where a woman is of childbearing age and sometimes where a patient is an elite or professional sportsperson.

Toxic drug warning

Some software includes a toxic drug warning for drugs where there is only a small difference between a therapeutic dose and a toxic dose. The warning might also remind you to check both the dose and the frequency. This can be very useful.

Spelling warning

Some software includes a warning when a drug being prescribed has a very similar spelling to another. This is a common source of error in prescriptions.

Compliance warning

Compliance warnings are based on the quantity and frequency of medication. While generally not useful for creams and skin preparations, they are reliable for pills and capsules. They can tell you if a patient has run out or is no longer taking a medication.

Progress notes

Progress notes can be the most difficult part of the computer medical record for a new user. You need to enter a considerable amount of data either during the course of the consultation or after it by referring to your handwritten notes. See Chapter 1 on computers and patient issues for advice on using the computer during the consultation.

WHAT IS THE BEST WAY OF TAKING NOTES?

Record your fully structured progress notes in fields that record specific information (e.g. weight, blood pressure, pulse or blood glucose).

Subjective information (history)

Generally, you will record the presenting complaint and patient issues as free text. Some packages have a structured, specific inquiry process, which may include questions about each organ system. You will be able to indicate that all responses were considered as 'no abnormality detected' (NAD). Make sure you ask all the questions. In a court of law, you may be asked specifically whether you asked each question in the software's inquiry process.

Some software allows quick access from this component of the medical record to other areas such as social and family history. This allows you to update one component of the health summary while still working in the progress notes. This avoids having to key sections of the medical record across multiple progress notes, as can happen in the paper record. In well-designed software, any changes you make to social or family history during this process will also be recorded in the notes, providing a track of that information as well as confirmation that the question was asked at that time.

Examination information
- Use free text carefully—you can't retrieve information in free text readily when trying to track important numbers or physical examination findings. You will also lose the capacity to use graphics.
- Become familiar with the checklists and the drawing tools, which are usually excellent.
- Take care in using features that allow the user to set a whole set of examination findings as NAD. If every one of the elements has not been examined do not use that tool.
- Some software allows you to add a digital camera image to the examination record. This is very useful for lacerations and skin lesions.

Reason for visit/diagnosis
Most diagnostic coding systems appropriate for general practice will incorporate symptoms as a reason/diagnosis. For example, 'lethargy' can be recorded as a reason or as a diagnosis.

When recording the reason for a visit, ask whether it is a one-off event or an ongoing health problem. This is important if the health problem is to appear in the health summary. Most packages allow this distinction. For example, you should treat the presentation and diagnosis of asthma as an ongoing health problem, but not for a simple upper respiratory tract infection.

Be aware that some packages retain a default position from patient to patient. If you set the default function to add a problem to the health summary of the last patient, this action will be retained when you see the next patient. This could result in an item being added to the same patient's record twice, or adding an item to a future patient's record unintentionally. You can delete the item, but it is time consuming.

Procedure
Enter data in the same way as recording a problem, as software will utilise the same coding or terminology dictionary. You will be able to perform quick audits and recalls for procedural issues.

Management plans

Using the computer saves time and results in a more complete record of your actions. The management plan builds up during the consultation—referrals and investigations are recorded. The software will also record any literature printed out from the patient information section.

When you come to write a management plan, simply note any additional matters discussed and advice given.

Review

You can record a review at the end of the consultation. You may also be able to post a recall, which will place a reminder in the main computer database. When the practice runs its regular recall, the reminder you have just posted will appear at the appropriate time.

Action list

Use an action list to remind yourself of things to consider at the next consultation, such as a breast examination. When you next open that patient's record, you will get a reminder.

This is a very handy tool which can be used for non-clinical matters such as reminding yourself to ask the patient about their recent holiday. They will think highly of you if they believe you can remember such details!

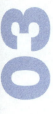

Abbreviations

Abbreviations are useful in special interest areas or as an aid to a regular management protocol. You can also choose abbreviations to use as a 'shortcut' (a set of brief keystrokes that enters a lengthy prewritten phrase into the progress notes).

Choose carefully to avoid common terms. For example, 'quit' might seem a good shortcut for 'giving up smoking, starting on patches today', but it will cause problems as this will appear every time you type 'quit'. Also, avoid obscure abbreviations that you may not remember.

PRACTICAL EXERCISE

Consider discussing how you enter progress notes with the other doctors in your practice or a small group, perhaps organised by your local division. One of the benefits of doing things within the practice is that you can create a solution that works for you. For example, you could discuss a 'shortcut'. Do you want to share the shortcuts with others in the practice, or restrict them to your own log-in profile?

Investigations

Computers are well suited to the simple repetitive task of investigations and offer major time savings to the GP and the practice.

HOW DO I ESTABLISH ELECTRONIC INVESTIGATION AND RESULT HANDLING?

The initial set-up is crucial. You might need to discuss your practice's needs with the software installation team.

Consider the following questions:

- Which pathology laboratories and imaging services does the practice use?
- For which of these services does the practice need to maintain pathology and radiology request forms in each consulting room?
- Which services accept electronic requests and is there an advantage in doing so?
- Which services will post electronic results to the practice?

This set-up process—including all the templates for pathology testing and imaging, with and without computer proprietary forms—can be time-consuming and tedious, but is very important.

Training is essential to ensure everyone in the practice knows how to:

- order investigations
- receive results
- undertake the reconciliation process
- hold results until the GP has indicated that they are free to be released to the patient record
- track outstanding results
- contact patients with their results.

HOW ELSE WILL THE COMPUTER HELP ME WITH INVESTIGATIONS?

Requests and ordering

This is straightforward. Click on an icon (pathology or imaging), choose a provider and the test, fill in the clinical details and print the request on the appropriate pathology or radiology form.

You can print requests on provider-supplied forms. Alternatively, get the computer to complete all the pathology testing and imaging details and generate a request on plain paper, so you don't have to keep a collection of stationery. The disadvantage is maintaining all the pathology testing and imaging details. This is particularly difficult with large or multiple pathology testing and imaging sites.

Selecting pathology tests and imaging requests

The selection of tests varies across packages. There will be tick boxes for short lists accompanied by a much more extensive list for all tests.

Some allow you to define a cluster of tests, such as might be required for a particular condition or examination.

You should be able to send a copy of the results to another doctor, which is useful for referrals. You may also be able to include the text from the current progress note, including the presenting complaint, on the request. However, be wary of cluttering the request with unnecessary detail. Either choose from a simple checklist or add your own brief clinical note. You could cut and paste relevant data from the progress note to the request. This is particularly useful in imaging requests.

Detailed check boxes allow you to set special information (e.g. pregnancy-related information, date of last period, fasting).

Processing results (electronic and scanning)

By receiving results electronically, you have a faster turnaround time and simpler handling and filing.

New results are stored in a holding area within the computer software. When you log in, you will be able to review all of your own results. You can then send a result straight to the record for filing with a simple key stroke. A recall for the next test can be posted and, where necessary, arrangements can be made to contact the patient.

It is important that your software can tell you when communication has failed. The computer can list tests for which results have not been received. Often this will be because the patient has not attended for the test. From a medicolegal viewpoint, you need to have a process that ensures that you are informed of the failure to complete the test and that the response of the doctor is recorded.

A cautionary note

Managing investigation requests and results is a matter of process. The computer offers excellent support for the routine process, but this can result in complacency. The computer is not good at managing the one-off event such as a patient choosing to go to an unusual pathology or radiology provider that is not flagged in the system.

Another difficulty which practices really need to work through is what to do with patients who do not have a test done. The computer does not automatically alert you to this. You also have to be very careful that once you have checked a result, the patient actually follows this up. While you might have a system for very abnormal test results, do you have a system which 'closes the loop' for results which are only mildly or moderately abnormal? What would happen if the patient failed to follow up in such cases? Would you know?

Managing the exceptions requires careful consideration. Your practice needs to consider and document how to integrate its procedures with the computer functions, including the management of exceptions.

Develop a protocol for downloading pathology and radiology results in your practice (in many practices this can be automated), when to check them and how patients should obtain their results (either in person or by phone). Most importantly, decide how to 'close the loop'—that is to ensure that should patients fail to enquire about their results, you will act on any significantly abnormal ones.

Immunisations

Immunisations and vaccinations are a separate but important component of the health summary. You should be able to look at any vaccine across the whole of the practice population in order to assess whether the practice is achieving a high enough level of vaccinations.

To record an immunisation select the immunisation from a list and then enter the balance of the data—the site given, the batch number and a comment to allow recording of any difficulty. The selection list is a component of the drug database and will be updated regularly with the prescribed medication list.

When adding vaccines, most software will remind you to check for allergies or other risks (e.g. pregnancy). This is helpful, but always check with the patient.

Immunisation software can remind you that a vaccine is due. Good software will search immunisation histories and add patients to the recall list when an immunisation is due. The procedure for handling recall information (automatic letter generation, phone recall) should be documented in the procedure manual.

Chronic disease management

As a practice develops a large pool of useful medical record information, a new world opens up in terms of disease management. For example, you can immediately communicate a new breakthrough in asthma management in children to all the parents of children in your practice with asthma. You can deal with an adverse reaction to a commonly used drug by generating a letter to all patients using the drug, instructing them how to proceed. General practice has been slow to take full advantage of these opportunities.

In recognition of this, the Australian Government has been building incentive systems around the use of computers in practice to improve the management of chronic disease. The immunisation incentive package is an example of how computers can alter the management of a health issue across the whole of Australia through general practice.

HOW CAN COMPUTERS HELP ME IMPROVE CHRONIC DISEASE MANAGEMENT?

The key to managing chronic disease and the associated incentive programs is maintaining a good health summary.

Managing asthma

Selecting a list of patients with asthma is a simple task in all software packages. Setting up recalls and regular follow-ups is equally simple. Some packages now offer the development and maintenance of asthma management plans. You can automatically retrieve data from the medication list, set the plan and print it for a patient in 20 to 30 seconds.

Managing diabetes

A number of packages include sophisticated diabetes monitoring tools. These combine all relevant information (e.g. blood sugars, glycated haemoglobin and referrals) to allow you to quickly review the progress of a diabetic patient and to take action where further tests or referrals are needed. A review that would otherwise take 5 to 10 minutes takes only 1 to 2 minutes on a computer.

Once this information is entered, the software can audit your performance with respect to diabetic patients. Your practice can set up appropriate recall strategies to improve that performance.

Health assessments

Health assessments are funded by Medicare for patients aged 75 years or more, and Aboriginal and Torres Strait Islander people aged 55 years or more. These assessments can take hours to complete. Some software packages have incorporated this assessment into the medical record program so that a trained nurse can easily complete the bulk of the data collection. It would then take only a few minutes more for you and the nurse to complete the recommendations.

If your practice has elderly patients, this is an essential tool.

GP management plans and team care arrangements

GP management plans and team care arrangements help you to improve the management of patients with chronic disease who require support from multiple health care providers. These plans record goals and review points, illustrating how relevant each problem is to patient management. The team care arrangements indicate the role of other health care providers in the medium-term management of patients with chronic and complex illnesses. Templates for these 'plans' are available through divisions of general practice. The use of templates is described in the next section.

This is a good example of how the computer record can generate complex information quickly and easily, assisting in patient management. It is not a feature of all software packages.

Letters and templates

You can format and type most of the referral letter, GP 'management plan' or 'team care arrangement' from a template on the computer, in less time than you could dictate it. All information available in the computer is placed in the relevant fields in the letter template.

You choose the recipient from the electronic address book and a letter is generated with their contact details. Patient record data is added from the health summary and the presenting complaint in the current progress note can be added to the letter—all done automatically. If desired you can add a couple of sentences before printing, faxing (this can be done directly via the computer system) or emailing the letter.

Involve the patient in this process by letting them check the letter on the screen. Ensure any special patient concerns or anxieties are reflected in the actual questions asked of the specialist (e.g. 'John is concerned that any shoulder surgery will preclude him playing squash').

HOW DO I CREATE REFERRAL LETTERS?

You will find it a simple task to set up the template to suit your style of referral letter. You can also add graphics such as a practice logo. Keep in mind that some graphic files are large and that storing this file with every letter created may use a considerable amount of hard disk space.

You may add more or less information from the health summary, according to your practice's style. Any block of information is readily available to use in the template.

HOW SHOULD I MANAGE LETTERS FROM SPECIALISTS?

Some specialists can email documents, which you can add to the record. Scan any letters on paper into the computer. Alternatively, type in a small summary and keep the original letter on file. Your practice should have systems in place where doctors are advised that a letter has been scanned and is ready for review before it is filed.

WHAT OTHER TEMPLATES ARE AVAILABLE?

Most packages have templates for sickness certificates, workers compensation certificates, health summaries, medication summaries and other documents. Software packages vary in how workers compensation certificates function, which may influence your choice of software.

REMEMBER!

Don't waste time designing your own templates when there is already one that would suit. Contact your division of general practice to see if others have produced a template that you might want.

PRACTICAL EXERCISE

Do you have electronic templates for health assessments, management plans and home medication reviews that work for you and your practice? Do you need to modify them? Again, it is not simply a case of having a form; you have to be able to use this in day-to-day practice. For example, preparing a 'team care arrangement' involves a number of stages, including: obtaining informed consent from the patient; establishing who is involved in the 'plan'; obtaining the input from the other health care providers; and discussing the final 'plan' with the patient at a subsequent consultation. The process is more difficult than the physical document! Have you established a manageable process?

Searches and audits

Most packages have reasonable search engines, but some are easier to use than others. The most flexible search engine tools are often the hardest to use as they rely on the user having some computer knowledge. The most user-friendly search tools have limited flexibility and facilitate the production of simple lists. Most software developers should be able to provide sophisticated search routines for special purposes, for a reasonable cost.

Two issues influence the capacity to go beyond the searches provided in your package: the underlying database tool and the actual structure of the data. Most modern software structures data in a format that facilitates searches of any element in the database.

Information in the demographics is the key to any search of the patient database. If an element such as 'occupation' is not recorded in a designated field, then you can't base a search on occupation.

HOW CAN I EXTRACT DATA?

Using the 'search databases' facility within the clinical software program enables you to develop lists of patients according to specific search criteria. However, what if you want to know what proportion of your patients who are being treated for hypertension have normalised blood pressures? Or the proportion of your patients with diabetes who have HbA1c levels less than or equal to 7.0?

Search tools within clinical software do not always allow you to make these kinds of enquiries, at least not currently. Software developers have developed 'extraction tools' which assist with this process, although their use remains limited at this stage.

WHY IS DATA ANALYSIS AND INTERPRETATION IMPORTANT?

The National Primary Care Collaboratives (NPCC), an Australian program based directly on a successful United Kingdom model, is a quality improvement program which emphasises how to make better use of clinical data. If you are interested in the details of the NPCC, you can visit its website at **www.npcc.com.au**

In broad terms, the program asks GPs to examine their data to see how closely they are following best practice guidelines. For example, in the case of diabetes, GPs are asked to investigate the percentage of patients with a last recorded:

- HbA1c of $\leq 7.0\%$
- cholesterol ≤ 4.0 mmol/L, and
- blood pressure of $\leq 130/80$.

Similarly, GPs are asked to document the percentage of patients with coronary heart disease who:

- are on aspirin
- are on a statin
- have had a myocardial infarction within the last 12 months and are on a beta blocker
- whose blood pressure is $\leq$ 140/90.

Various data extraction tools can be used to aggregate this information at the practice level. What can you do with the data? By comparing your practice with others in the region, you will see whether you are following clinical guidelines as well as other practices. The aim is not to get 100 per cent of patients reaching clinical targets; this would be unrealistic for a number of reasons. The principal aim is for your figures to improve until you reach 'best practice'.

You can discuss your data within your practice at one of your regular meetings, or you might find that your division of general practice can provide you with feedback. You will then need to consider carefully how 'quality improvement' strategies can help your practice better meet clinical targets.

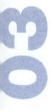

GPs in the United Kingdom receive financial incentives to meet a range of clinical targets. This is described in a little more detail in Chapter 6. Clinical data analysis does of course mean that GPs need to be conscientious in entering data in the first place.

The chief beneficiaries of this audit process are your patients. You would therefore do this without additional financial incentives, wouldn't you? Mind you, GPs who impress on patients that computers can be used to improve health might have a marketing advantage. There could be something in it for GPs as well!

PRACTICAL EXERCISE

Perform a simple audit to see if your practice has a complete set of health data for the majority of your patients. Nominate a session to do the audit, and record whether consecutive patients for that session have the following basic information recorded:

- up-to-date drug list
- drug allergies
- past history list.

At your next practice meeting, discuss the results of the audit and how you can improve the completeness of the basic health data.

Recalls and reminders

Recalls and reminders have already been covered, but it is important to elaborate on the definitions of the two tools.

A reminder is a patient-based tool; it is opportunistic. When a patient attends and the medical record is open, a reminder indicates an issue that might need to be considered in this particular consultation.

A recall is an active process. When the date of the recall arrives, an alert is posted to a list for use in active recall (e.g. recall letters or telephone recall). At the same time a reminder is posted in the patient's medical record in case they attend before the recall. You can automatically generate a recall by applying a protocol, for example 'all men aged more than 50 years should have a recall for faecal occult blood testing'. As each male patient reaches an age of 50 years, the recall will be posted to the recall list and a reminder to the patient record.

You can generate a recall for an individual patient or across a group of patients after a search of the database.

A recall should always have a date of recall and a reason. You can choose the reason from a checklist or create it in free text. When recalls remain unattended past their due date, you can quickly assess the importance of the recall.

You can complete a recall or reminder at the time of a consultation by simply deleting or resetting the date. It is important to undertake this clearing process. Your practice should develop a protocol for dealing with outstanding recalls. The doctor or nurse should first check the medical record and confirm the patient has not attended, and is still with the practice.

PRACTICAL EXERCISE

The computer is a tool enabling you to keep track of when people need to be reminded about a follow-up clinical intervention. If you have not already done so, start with recalls and reminders for a single condition (e.g. Pap tests). Once this process is established, you can consider applying it to other clinical areas, such as conditions that cause the most preventable morbidity and mortality in your practice area. Establish a protocol for running the system (e.g. who enters the data, who sends out recall letters and who follows up with the patient). What safeguards have been taken to ensure that if patients notify you of a change of address, the practice recall database will be updated?

Decision support tools

As you incorporate medical records into a sophisticated software system, you will be able to access more-relevant information as you work.

WHAT DECISION SUPPORT TOOLS CAN I EXPECT TO FIND IN THE COMPUTER?

The first generation of decision support tools lived outside the medical record software. The software package 'Therapeutic Guidelines' (see **www.tg.com.au**) is a very good example of a sophisticated decision support tool. However, you cannot easily move information from a particular progress note to the separate decision support tool. For example, if you are seeing a patient with ankylosing spondylitis and looking for therapeutic options, you will have to move to the other software and enter 'ankylosing spondylitis' as a search term. The ideal solution would be for the computer record to automatically offer the list of therapeutic options when you enter the problem in the progress note.

The drug database that exists within the medical record software demonstrates the benefits of decision support at the time of prescribing. In time, this concept of integration will extend to all elements of diagnosis, investigation and management.

The key to good decision support is having relevant information offered at the time you, the GP, needs it.

Poor decision support software may alert you to irrelevant information too often. If you are constantly reminded of a problem that is irrelevant to most of your patients, you may be inclined to switch off the alert or ignore it by the time a patient arrives who is concerned with that problem.

WHAT ABOUT UPDATING SUPPORT INFORMATION?

Updating decision support information is a major challenge. This is particularly true where a number of separate packages are used in addition to the medical record. Loading three to four updates each month from different sources is time consuming and inefficient.

The best way would be automatic updating from the Internet. Broadband Internet access makes it feasible to have a considerable amount of the support information directly available from the Internet, rather than having it on the computer on the desk. This will allow regular, reliable updating provided at a relatively low cost to users.

In the future, we will see increasing integration of decision support software and medical record software. As the structure of the record becomes more reliable, the additional decision support software will become more sophisticated.

You can find further information about decision support in Chapter 4 on electronic resources.

Summary

Most practices adopt their clinical software in stages. The biggest change is when the consultation 'progress notes' replace paper-based health records. You need to be ready to adopt this change.

User skills also come in stages. This is largely about using the computer as part of a broader 'system' within the practice, such as handling pathology results or using the computer to assist with chronic disease management. It is important to have a good understanding of the basics first, rather than trying to do too much all at once. For example, simply keeping drug lists, allergies and past history information up-to-date is crucial if other aspects of the computer are to function properly. Without basic data entry, the computer is no better than the passive paper record.

Change in this area requires repeated attempts to develop efficient routines in using your computer.

Electronic resources

You do not need a high degree of computer skill to benefit from using electronic resources in general practice, but you do need to understand some key points of computer-based searches. This chapter provides some tips to help you use electronic resources, including the Internet, to find evidence-based information.

This chapter will help develop your search skills so you can have credible, relevant information when you need it, and have the confidence to use these resources in your clinical practice.

CONTENTS

When you have completed this chapter, you should be able to:

- define the clinical problem you want to answer
- list different sources of information and resources to help answer clinical queries
- define 'levels of evidence' for published clinical information
- decide when the Internet is useful in clinical practice
- conduct an Internet search for clinical information
- identify useful Internet resources and websites
- select the best evidence from Internet sources
- judge the quality and relevance of the information
- confidently incorporate the use of the Internet into your consultation with patients
- use the Internet to enhance patient care.

Introduction

As a GP, you aim to use relevant and high-quality clinical information. Applying it with patients is the foundation of evidence-based practice.

Chapter 3 explained how to use clinical software to help with your consultation, but your clinical software may not always have the answers you need. For example, you might not know how to interpret a test result.

This chapter describes how you can use your computer to access other resources and find the answers. Electronic resources include CD-ROMs and specialised software, but the main focus of this chapter is on how to find information using the Internet.

Take this progression in steps. Become familiar with a few websites first, and then gain wider experience as you become more confident.

Using electronic resources

WHY USE ELECTRONIC INFORMATION RESOURCES?

The amount of medical knowledge doubles every 19 years. General practitioners face a constant stream of updates about clinical medicine and practice management. How can you keep up-to-date, and how can you recall that pertinent fact when you need it?

There are a number of options. You could:

- look up the answer in a textbook
- attend a clinical update meeting

- talk to a medical specialist
- telephone a reputable advisory body such as the National Prescribing Service's Therapeutic Advice and Information Service (TAIS; see **www.nps.org.au**)
- look for the information yourself in any one of the electronic resources accessible via your computer.

If you are using clinical record or prescribing software, you will find many answers integrated into these programs, such as approved drug product information, drug interaction tables and immunisation schedules. You can also subscribe to other electronic resources and install them on your computer. For example, you can find electronic versions of *Therapeutic Guidelines* at **www.tg.com.au**, and the *Australian Medicines Handbook* at **www.amh.net.au**

Other useful sources of best practice information freely available over the Internet include the *Australian Immunisation Handbook* 8th edition (National Health and Medical Research Council 2003), the Royal College of Pathologists of Australasia's (RCPA) *Manual of the Use and Interpretation of Pathology Tests*, the NPS RADAR program (which is also incorporated into a number of GP prescribing packages) and the Cochrane Library.

Australian Family Physician, *The Medical Journal of Australia*, *Australian Prescriber* and the *British Medical Journal* (BMJ) are also available online, and you can use Internet search engines to access the major journal repositories such as the MEDLINE database. The United Kingdom's National Health Service (NHS) has collected many useful resources together into a national electronic library for health (at **www.nelh.nhs.uk**) which can be accessed by registered medical practitioners.

Broadband Internet access will make it faster and easier to search during working hours. Australian GPs can check out the Australian Government's Broadband for Health Programme (**www.health.gov.au/internet/wcms/publishing.nsf/Content/health-ehealth-broadband-initiative.htm**) to obtain recommendations on suitable Internet service providers.

In the future, you can expect to have many electronic knowledge resources available on your desktop computer via the web, and decision support software capable of two-way communication with knowledge providers and electronic medical record repositories.

Active methods of accessing information also mean you are more likely to retain it, and be able to apply it again in a clinical setting. When you seek evidence-based solutions to patient problems during the consultation, it provides an opportunity to involve and educate the patient. You could also direct them to useful websites, especially if they have a chronic disease.

WHERE WILL I FIND THE INFORMATION?

There are different sources of knowledge available through electronic resources, often described as the information hierarchy (Figure 4.1).

FIGURE 4.1 INFORMATION HIERARCHY

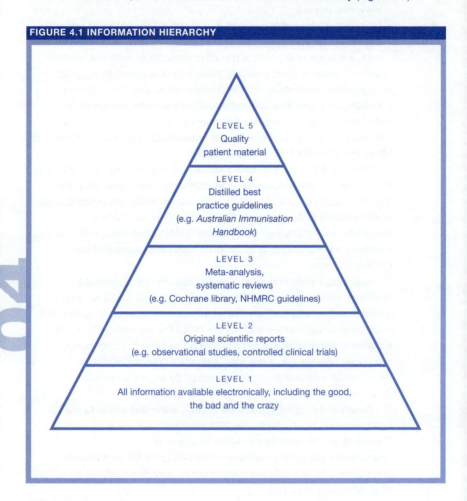

LEVEL 5
Quality
patient material

LEVEL 4
Distilled best
practice guidelines
(e.g. *Australian Immunisation
Handbook*)

LEVEL 3
Meta-analysis,
systematic reviews
(e.g. Cochrane library, NHMRC guidelines)

LEVEL 2
Original scientific reports
(e.g. observational studies, controlled clinical trials)

LEVEL 1
All information available electronically, including the good,
the bad and the crazy

- Level one contains all the information available electronically on any one topic. There are no filters here to weed out the good from the bad.
- Level two consists of original research reports in peer-reviewed journals. The volume of information makes it impossible to find quick answers to practical questions. It is important to make sure you are looking at the latest results, as these can contradict earlier clinical trials.

- Level three consists of meta-analyses and systematic reviews. They attempt to distill relevant information from good-quality clinical trials and provide evidence-based overviews of particular topics. These can be useful for particular questions but a lot of information must be sorted through to find what you're looking for.
- Level four consists of authoritative, comprehensive but succinct best practice clinical guidelines. Australian examples take into account local practice (such as drugs available on the Pharmaceutical Benefits Scheme) as well as the evidence available from meta-analyses, systematic reviews and original research articles. A number of authoritative international medical textbooks are also available electronically.
- Level five contains quality information based on knowledge extracted from the previous levels but written in user-friendly language. One electronic example for consumer information on health and diseases is available from the government-sponsored HealthInsite (see Table 4.7).

You will learn through practise and experience when to use electronic resources for clinical information, and which electronic resources are more helpful than others. You will gain some experience by working through the case studies later in the chapter.

Useful electronic resources

This section provides a series of tables listing useful electronic resources and some tips for using them. Some of these sites will require a subscription or licence fee for certain prescribing software. If the site does not mention a charge, assume that use of the site is free.

> **REMEMBER!**
> You will find answers in a variety of sources, but use 'authoritative' ones if you can. They are likely to be the most relevant to your clinical practice.

Table 4.1 shows sites for Australian best practice guidelines or similar. The list is not comprehensive; there are many other useful resources. All these resources are compiled by Australian teams of experts and updated regularly.

TABLE 4.1 AUSTRALIAN BEST PRACTICE GUIDELINES OR SIMILAR		
Name	**Website address**	**Comments**
Australian Immunisation Handbook	www9.health.gov.au/ immhandbook	Current Australian immunisation recommendations; good patient material.
Australian Medicines Handbook	www.amh.net.au	Independent drug monographs organised by organ system and therapeutic class, featuring comparative information about different drugs within the same class. A better educational resource and more up-to-date than approved product information. Subscription required.
Therapeutic Guidelines	www.tg.com.au	Independent disease/problem-oriented guidelines giving practical and succinct drug and non-drug recommendations for therapy. Subscription required.
Pharmaceutical Benefits Schedule (PBS)	www.pbs.gov.au/ html/home	Up-to-date list of government-subsidised drugs including notes and cautions.
National Prescribing Service	www.nps.org.au www.npsradar.org.au	Excellent therapeutic resources including fact sheets, case studies, clinical audits and information about new PBS drugs (RADAR reviews), with email alerts available.
RCPA Manual	www.rcpamanual.edu.au	Extensive and useful information about laboratory tests; can also be entered by clinical problem. Indexing and searching needs improvement. Some educational case scenarios.
The RACGP Red Book	www.racgp.org.au/ redbook	Guidelines for preventive activities in general practice, also available as a downloadable file.

Table 4.2 shows some sites that provide meta-analyses and systematic reviews.

TABLE 4.2 META-ANALYSIS AND SYSTEMATIC REVIEWS		
Name	**Website address**	**Comments**
The Cochrane Library	www.thecochranelibrary. org	A collection of excellent systematic reviews. It also provides graphical summaries of its meta-analyses (forest plots) showing odds, ratios and numbers needed to treat (with confidence intervals).
Clinical evidence	www.clinicalevidence.com	BMJ evidence-based reviews on common clinical problems. Subscription required.
NHS Centre for Reviews and Dissemination	www.york.ac.uk/inst/crd	Various databases and publications mainly in downloadable files.

Table 4.3 lists websites for electronic textbooks and guidelines. Other textbooks, such as *Harrisons Online*, come bundled with subscriptions to clinical software. These e-books have not been included in this table.

TABLE 4.3 ELECTRONIC TEXTBOOKS AND GUIDELINES

Name	Website address	Comments
Merck Manuals	www.merck.com/ mrkshared/mmanual/ home.jsp	*The Merck Manual of Diagnosis and Therapy*, 2004
GPnotebook	www.gpnotebook.co.uk/ homepage.cfm	A United Kingdom general practice textbook.
National Guideline Clearinghouse	www.guideline.gov	United States Department of Health and Human Services' site.
NHMRC guidelines	www.nhmrc.gov.au/ publications/index.htm	Systematic reviews of topical subjects, mainly available in downloadable files.
New Zealand Guidelines Group	http://www.nzgg.org.nz	A very comprehensive site for clinical practice guidelines.

Table 4.4 lists relevant electronic journals, bulletins and newspapers. Several of these resources provide email alerting services to notify you of a journal's latest issue's table of contents (TOC), or articles relevant to a specific area of interest that you nominate.

TABLE 4.4 ELECTRONIC JOURNALS, BULLETINS AND NEWSPAPERS

Name	Website address	Comments
The Medical Journal of Australia	www.mja.com.au	General interest medical topics; some practice guidelines.
British Medical Journal (BMJ)	www.bmj.com	International in scope; many useful articles for GPs; topic collections available; good search engine; TOC and topic alerts. Subscription required for full contents.
Australian Family Physician	www.racgp.org.au/ publications/afp_ online.asp	General practice focused; new online version being developed; has clinical challenge questions.
Australian Prescriber	www.australian prescriber.com	Australia's independent drug bulletin aimed at doctors, dentists, pharmacists and students.
Australian Doctor	www.australiandoctor. com.au	Medicopolitical news and useful links.
Medical Observer	www.medicalobserver. com.au	Medicopolitical news and useful links.

Table 4.5 contains a list of medical databases, as well as search engines that can be used for medical and general purposes.

TABLE 4.5 MEDICAL DATABASES, MEDICAL AND GENERAL PURPOSE SEARCH ENGINES

Name	Website address	Comments
MEDLINE via PubMed	www.pubmed.com	Abstracts of research papers, reviews and guidelines; some links to full text articles.
ProQuest	www.racgp.org.au/library	Many full text articles (for RACGP members only).
SUMSearch	sumsearch.uthscsa.edu	Searches MEDLINE, guidelines and textbooks.
HONSelect	www.hon.ch	Search integrator for medical and health queries.
Intute	www.intute.ac.uk/ healthandlifesciences/ medicine	This site, formerly called Organising Medical Networked Information (OMNI), presents both health professional and consumer information.
Medical Matrix	www.medmatrix.org/reg/ login.asp	Excellent site; requires a subscription.
Google	www.google.com.au	General search engine; can be very useful, but searches are likely to return some irrelevant results.

A number of institutions such as universities use the browser MEDLINE via Ovid. They pay a fee on behalf of their students and staff, making a large number of full text articles available at no charge to individual users.

Other search engines try to find answers by searching several medical databases (the 'one-stop shop' approach). This includes the Unified Search Environment which is used in Australia by Health Communication Network and its clinical package, Medical Director (USEMD). Subscribers can access USEMD from within the clinical software program. This search engine uses a more intuitive approach than MEDLINE.

Most clinical software packages also contain a selection of useful calculators. You can also find a wide range of online calculators (with links to other related resources) at http://emedicine.com/etools/index.htm

The Internet is also useful for continuing your medical education. Table 4.6 lists some useful sites.

TABLE 4.6 CONTINUING MEDICAL EDUCATION

Name	Website address	Comments
gplearning	www.gplearning.gpea. com.au	Has interactive education activities and is accredited for continuing professional development points.
Omnus	www.omnus.com.au	Has continuing professional development points.
PriMeD	www.primed.com.au	Has continuing professional development points.
bmjlearning	www.bmjlearning.com	Provided by the *British Medical Journal*; requires subscription.

Some sites contain quality consumer information and allow patients to maintain their own records. Table 4.7 lists some of these.

TABLE 4.7 QUALITY CONSUMER INFORMATION, SELF-MAINTAINED PATIENT RECORDS

Name	Website address	Comments
Informed Health Online	www.informedhealthonline. org/index.en.html	Promotes consumer accessibility of health information from the Cochrane Collaboration.
HealthInsite	www.healthinsite.gov.au	Australian Government consumer site which provides information leaflets on a variety of clinical conditions.
Better Health Channel	www.betterhealth.vic. gov.au	Victorian Government consumer site, with similar resources to HealthInsite.
National Prescribing Service	www.nps.org.au	Medimate helps consumers keep track of their medicines; Medicines Line (telephone 1300 888 763) provides independent, accurate, up-to-date information about medicines.
MEDLINEPlus	http://medlineplus.gov	Based in the United States, this government site provides medical articles for consumers.
MIMS myDr	www.mydr.com.au	Health information, calculators and quizzes; self-maintained patient record; contains a comprehensive set of consumer medicines information.

Portals attempt to provide a 'one-stop shop' to many relevant medical resources. Table 4.8 lists some useful medical portals.

TABLE 4.8 MEDICAL PORTALS

Name	Website address	Comments
Drs Reference Site	www.drsref.com.au	Australian site; useful links and e-textbooks; requires registration.
National Electronic Library for Health	www.nelh.nhs.uk	United Kingdom NHS site; aims to provide clinicians with access to the best current knowledge to support health care related decisions.
Medic8®	www.medic8.com/ index.htm	United Kingdom site with useful clinical resources, including e-textbooks; content reviewed by 'a qualified UK doctor'.
AusDoctors.net	www.ausdoctors.net	Australian portal with educational and information resources
Medscape	www.medscape.com	United States medical portal; news and continuing medical education site.

Table 4.9 contains a small sample of the many other useful sites.

TABLE 4.9 OTHER USEFUL SITES		
Name	Website address	Comments
Centre for Evidence-Based Medicine (EBM)	www.cebm.net/index.asp	Excellent site to learn, do and teach about EBM; also has EBM tools.
National Heart Foundation	www.heartfoundation. com.au	Cardiovascular guidelines and consumer information.
International Diabetes Institute	www.idi.org.au	Good consumer fact sheets.
Centres for Disease Control and Prevention travel site	www.cdc.gov/travel	United States' created information for travel health.
World Health Organisation (WHO) International Travel and Health	www.who.int/ith/en/	WHO travel site.
DermIS	http://dermis.multimedica. de/index_e.html	Browse over 4500 dermatology images online.

Clinical decision support systems

WHAT DOES A CLINICAL DECISION SUPPORT SYSTEM DO?

A clinical decision support system compares patient characteristics with a credible knowledge base and then offers specific advice. It incorporates evidence-based guidelines and a summary of patient data, which helps your clinical decision making.

Decision support is classified by the following levels of increasing complexity:
- narrative decision support
- active decision support
- algorithmic decision support.

Narrative decision support
This accesses electronic resources through links in the clinical software. The electronic resources operate in isolation but are more readily accessed than stand-alone programs installed on the electronic desktop (or CD-ROMs).

Active decision support
These electronic resources link more intimately with your clinical software. For example, when you select a drug to prescribe, you receive best practice recommendations at the click of a button. The NPS RADAR program (information about new PBS drugs) is an example of this type of decision support. In this case, information is provided on your screen automatically when certain new drugs are prescribed.

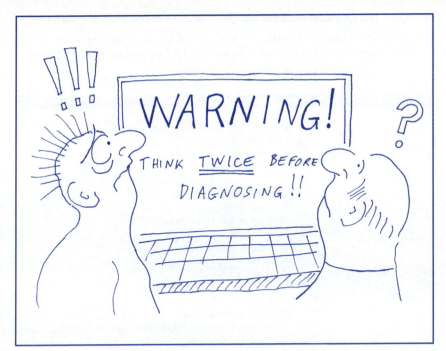

The latest indecision support tool

Algorithmic decision support
This third level of integration generates succinct, patient-specific recommendations for clinical decisions and action based on data contained in the patient electronic medical record and guideline/handbook recommendations. This level of decision support exists in drug allergy, drug and drug, and drug and disease interaction checks carried out by most prescribing packages.

WHAT ARE THE LIMITATIONS OF DECISION SUPPORT SYSTEMS?

Decision support systems have some limitations.
- It is important that key data such as the patient's allergy status, current drug history and breastfeeding status, be entered into the system.
- Different prescribing packages respond differently to a standard set of drug to drug interactions. You may miss important interactions if you become desensitised after too many alerts.
- Australian clinical software packages need external validation of decision support capabilities.
- More research is required on how best to provide succinct and relevant computerised decision support to busy GPs.

The capability of prescribing software packages varies. Check with software vendors to find out what the software can do. Table 4.10 lists some of the clinical support tools available.

TABLE 4.10 CLINICAL SUPPORT RESOURCES	
Area	Resources
Medication	Drug database by brand and generic names
	Approved product information
	Consumer product information (CPI)
	RADAR (information on new PBS listings)
	Drug to drug interaction warning
	Drug allergy warning
	Drug disease warning
	Drug use in pregnancy information
	Drug breastfeeding warning
Immunisation	Australian immunisation schedule
	Immunisation management/history/reminders
Clinical tools/calculators	Coronary risk calculator
	Estimated date of delivery calculator
	Dose calculator
	Metric conversion calculator
	Ideal weight/body mass index/body surface area calculator
	Paediatric growth charts
	Respiratory function calculator
	Creatinine clearance
Travel	Country risk information
	Vaccination database
	Patient leaflets
Other	Patient recall/screening
	Report generation
	Medicare schedule
	Prevention activities
	Patient educational material
	Pathology result viewing
	Templates for referrals
	Physical activity monitor

Tips on searching for information

HOW CAN I FIND THE INFORMATION I NEED?

The first step is to decide the reason for your search. Do you want to find out what is interesting or new?

• Search an electronic journal. Remember, most offer an alert service to keep you up-to-date.

• Go to a specific site for continuing medication education.

Do you need to find the answer to a specific clinical question?
- Search in a set of comprehensive best practice clinical guidelines (Figure 4.1, level 4).
- If you don't find the information there then use SUMSearch to check the Cochrane Library (Figure 4.1, level 3).
- Failing that, search medical databases of original articles (Figure 4.1, level 2).

Quality patient information (Figure 4.1, level 5) is usually found on the specific websites listed in Table 4.1.

REMEMBER!

Become familiar with a small number of resources rather than trying to use too many.

Practice and experience will teach you when to use electronic resources for clinical information, which Internet sites are more helpful than others, and how to find the information you need.

REMEMBER!

Set up a list of 'bookmarks' or 'favourites' for your most used Internet sites, and group them in a logical order. You could use the websites in the previous tables to establish a useful set of bookmarks.

Develop a structured clinical question
A structured question will help to clarify what you really want to know. It will also make you think about the search words you will use, particularly for the large medical databases such as MEDLINE and the meta-search engine SUMSearch.

Structure your questions as precisely as possible. For example, instead of asking 'Are antibiotics any good for acute bronchitis?', a more useful form might be 'In patients with acute bronchitis, does the use of antibiotics lead to a reduction in the duration of cough compared with not using antibiotics?'.

The PICO (Patient, Intervention, Comparator, Outcome) format is a common way of structuring a search question. The following example involves the intuitive question 'Are antibiotics any good for acute bronchitis?':

P   Patient

        Patient population in question (acute bronchitis patients)

I   Intervention

        The treatment or intervention being measured (antibiotics)

C   Comparator

        Effect of the intervention in comparison to what (no antibiotics)

O   Outcome

        The outcome to be achieved (duration of cough)

Extract the key search terms from the question. Remember to allow for different spellings and regional variations. For example, hypercholesterolaemia may also be referred to as hyperlipidemia, and have different spellings.

The PICO format will also help you to consider synonyms for the search terms. For example, you might want to search for patients with 'lower respiratory tract infection' as well as 'acute bronchitis'.

Some questions will not contain each of these components and you don't have to use all of them as search terms. For example, it is unlikely that you will use the word 'cough' as a search term as it is a common term and will return many results. This structured approach is less relevant for the more subject specific sites.

Some databases ask specifically for the type of question or the focus of the question. MEDLINE (see the clinical queries section of PubMed) and SUMSearch have focus radio buttons.

Use Boolean operators when searching
You have your structured question. Now you need to think about where to look for an answer. Generic search skills will be useful, but search techniques vary from site to site. Refer to the sections on MEDLINE, SUMSearch and Cochrane in this chapter for specific tips.

The search techniques described below are most useful for medical databases such as MEDLINE and the Cochrane Library, and search engines such as SUMSearch and Google. Details will vary, but the same principles apply when conducting a search using:
- connecting words (Boolean operators)
- word stems (truncation)
- a thesaurus (MeSH terms).

Boolean operators are the words 'AND', 'OR' and 'NOT'. They are used to combine or exclude terms.
- 'AND' requires both terms to be present (e.g. stroke AND hypertension).
- 'OR' requires at least one term to be present (e.g. hypercholesterolaemia OR hyperlipidaemia).
- 'NOT' excludes the second term (e.g. asthma NOT children).

Boolean operators can be case sensitive. When in doubt, write them in upper-case letters. This also differentiates them from the search terms.

Truncation refers to shortening a word to its stem. It has few disadvantages (unless the stem word becomes ambiguous) and enables a more inclusive search. Use it whenever you can. For example, enter 'myocard*' to search for any words beginning with these letters, such as myocardial, myocardium and myocarditis. Some databases require a 'wild card' for truncation, with most using the * symbol. In some databases, truncation is automatic (i.e. you don't need to use symbols); in the previous example you would simply enter 'myocard'.

MeSH (medical subject headings) refers to a list of vocabulary terms that classify the subjects of medical articles. For example, papers about raised blood pressure are classified under 'hypertension' rather than 'high blood pressure'. It is the official dictionary of databases, and is particularly associated with MEDLINE.

The alternative to using MeSH terms is to use free text. It is often better to use both systems. Generally, MeSH is more accurate. When a MeSH term is used, it automatically searches all of the subheadings.

MeSH terms reflect the subject, population, nature of study, publication type, and so on, of the paper they classify. To find the appropriate MeSH term for a word or phrase, search the MeSH dictionary on databases such as MEDLINE.

To answer a specific clinical question, conduct a search in one of the large databases or medical search engines. The list in Table 4.11 is a good place to start. Structure your question first and then think about possible search terms.

TABLE 4.11 LARGE DATABASES AND MEDICAL SEARCH ENGINES

Search engine/database	Search method	Search operators
SUMSEARCH Majority of links come from: • the Cochrane Library, including DARE (Database of Abstracts of Reviews of Effectiveness) reviews that have been produced outside the Cochrane Collaboration itself • MEDLINE (PubMed) • National Guidelines Clearinghouse (a United States site). A search is twice as likely to succeed if you include no more than two words within each search entry, and use a MeSH heading.	Combines metasearching with contingency searching: • metasearching means searching multiple databases and then collating the results • contingency searching means searching with intelligence (i.e. when a search returns an excessive number of results, SUMSearch will execute a more restrictive search until you have an optimal number of hits; too few hits will see it search another site to find more results).	• Boolean operators. • Truncation symbols $ or *.

(cont. overleaf)

Search engine/database	Search method	Search operators
COCHRANE LIBRARY An international network of clinicians, academics and consumers. It includes: • systematic reviews • database of other systematic reviews (DARE) • register of controlled trials. Cochrane reviews are mainly about the effects of health care. They are highly structured and systematic and evidence is included or excluded according to explicit quality criteria to minimise bias.	Allows you to: • browse the abstracts in alphabetical order or conduct a search • start your search with general topics (e.g. asthma). The database is not large so you can easily browse through all the papers on a topic.	• Boolean operators are no applicable. • Truncation is automatic.
PUBMED Web-based retrieval system developed at the National Library of Medicine in Washington: • database of bibliographic information drawn from the life sciences literature (database is called MEDLINE) • includes over 4000 journals and 11 million records, dating back to 1966 • access is free but most papers are in abstract form only.	Search through: • main page • clinical queries feature, which uses built-in filters within given categories (therapy, diagnosis, aetiology or prognosis). You can search with high sensitivity (more results with some less relevant) or high specificity (a more precise search, but you might miss some articles). Allows searches for systematic reviews only.	• Supports upper-case Boolean operators (AND, OR, NOT). • Truncation by the symbol *.
GOOGLE As in other search engines, you need to consider: • synonyms (e.g. heart disease and cardiac disease) • acronyms (e.g. ESR and erythrocyte sedimentation rate) • singular or plural forms (e.g. woman and women) • variations in spelling (e.g. oesophagus and esophagus).	Google also has an advanced search facility that helps you to either narrow or broaden your search.	• Uses the + and – signs as its Boolean symbols. • Does not allow truncation. • Does not specifically use MeSH terms.

HOW CAN I JUDGE THE QUALITY OF CLINICAL INFORMATION RETRIEVED?

You need information that is valid and relevant. Critical appraisal methods are beyond the scope of this module, but you can assess the quality of the information by considering:

• the reputation of the site
• when the material was last updated
• who wrote the material
• in which journal it was published
• who, if anyone, reviewed the material

- which institution supported the authors
- whether conflicts of interest are declared
- whether the site has achieved official sanction; for example, by the Health On the Net (HON) Foundation.

You could try to judge the quality (internal validity) of research papers yourself through critical appraisal. You can use checklists of appraisal criteria to judge the quality of experimental and observational studies, systematic reviews and clinical practice guidelines. However, critical appraisal is beyond the scope of this module, and most GPs would also find it very difficult unless they had done postgraduate study in the field.

HOW DO I APPLY RESEARCH EVIDENCE TO INDIVIDUAL PATIENTS?

A research paper tells you the outcome of an average person in a study, but the relevance of a study to other individuals depends on the external validity of the study. Bear in mind that:
- patients are rarely 'average'
- their characteristics may not match those of the patients in the study
- the results may not be entirely reliable.

Many research papers try to quantify the probability of benefit. The number needed to treat (NNT) is a useful statistic that refers to the number of people who need to be treated before there is one person who benefits (or avoids an adverse outcome). For example, one might need to treat 50 people with hypertension for 5 years to prevent one stroke. In this case, the NNT is 50.

You can use evidence directly in your consultations. For example, a Cochrane review on otitis media shows that you need to treat nine children with antibiotics before one will benefit. You can use this information to help patients (or, in this case, their parents) decide whether they want antibiotics or not. But finding relevant and credible clinical information on the Internet is only one part of the decision-making process. You need to take into account the patient's wishes and values, and consider what is affordable and available.

HOW DO I IMPROVE MY ABILITY TO SEARCH FOR AND APPLY EVIDENCE?

The best way to improve your search skills, increase your familiarity with various websites and understand the range of information available is to practise. There is no better way.

Practise searching while you try to answer questions that arise in your own practice. Discuss your techniques with other GPs or set up a journal club, where GPs take turns in finding answers to clinical questions.

You can seek help from librarians at the RACGP (for college members), hospital librarians and possibly your local division of general practice. Academic departments of general practice can also assist, and are particularly helpful if you wish to increase your skills in critical appraisal.

Solving case studies using electronic resources

The following four case studies demonstrate how to use electronic resources to solve practical problems. The first example uses a general medical search engine; the others involve specific resources.

Case study **4.1**

Should children with mild croup be given oral steroids?

Where to start?

SUMSearch is a logical place to start. It searches multiple databases and collates the results. This search engine could be called a metasearch engine of evidence-based sites.

If you enter the search terms 'croup' and the truncated 'steroid*' (which includes the plural form), you end up with forty-five 'hits'. These include:

- two reviews found in the Cochrane Library
- four possible systematic reviews and thirty-nine other articles in PubMed.

It is possible to have a look at the article headings and summaries to see which articles are worth reading in more detail—this may only be one or two from the forty-five hits. Always aim to find the most authoritative and recent form of evidence. In this case it would be one of the systematic reviews in the Cochrane Library.

The most relevant paper is in the DARE collection within the Cochrane Library. This refers to the evidence on the benefits of steroids for moderate to severe croup. Decide whether you can therefore apply this to the milder cases seen in general practice.

Case study **4.2**

Should a child aged 4 years have the meningococcal vaccine?

Where to start?

The obvious place to go is the *Australian Immunisation Handbook* 8th Edition (2003), available online at **www9.health.gov.au/immhandbook**

The index indicates some relevant information. Clicking on this index item provides an answer to the question asked.

This site also contains excellent information for parents in a variety of languages, which can be printed off to reinforce advice given.

Case study **4.3**

A male aged 40 years, feeling unwell on lithium

A male aged 40 years with bipolar disorder controlled by lithium (slow release preparation 450mg taken every 12 hours) presents feeling tired, weak and shaky, and complaining of nausea. The patient is taking plasma lithium, 1.6 mmol/L; taken 8 hours after the last dose (therapeutic range for chronic maintenance 0.6 to 1.2 mmol/L). The patient is also taking ibuprofen. What are the causes of lithium toxicity?

Where to start?

The Royal College of Pathologists of Australasia (RCPA) *Manual of the Use and Interpretation of Pathology Tests*, available at **www.rcpamanual.edu.au**, seems a sensible place to start.

However, there are some drawbacks to this resource. The specific search for 'lithium toxicity' produces no hits. A general search for 'lithium' produces a large number of apparently irrelevant hits.

It's a convoluted process to find information about lithium testing, but you can follow a series of links to the information: From 'Pathology tests', go to 'Complete pathology test listing', then 'Pathology tests' by alphabetical order, 'L', 'Lithium', 'Lithium serum'.

Having followed this path, the information provided on increased levels is not helpful (increased levels may occur in sodium depletion; for example, associated with diuretics).

Although this electronic manual has some excellent information, its search function needs more work.

Another search is conducted for 'lithium toxicity' in the electronic version of *Therapeutic Guidelines* (eTG complete), available on subscription from **www.tg.com.au**

The results indicate that the patient's lithium toxicity is the result of the patient's self administration of ibuprofen, a non-steroidal anti-inflammatory drug (NSAID). Information provided at the site notes that serum lithium concentrations are increased by all NSAIDs (except sulindac and aspirin) and suggests either using another analgesic or reducing the lithium dose by 30 to 50 per cent and monitoring serum lithium concentrations closely. Similar information can be found in the electronic version of the *Australian Medicines Handbook* (available by subscription at **www.amh.net.au**) and from the drug interaction section of approved product information.

Case study **4.4**

A male aged 20 years, with a dog bite—does he need antibiotics?

A male aged 20 years presents with several lacerations on his hand from a dog bite (sustained 30 minutes ago). You recommend antibiotics but he is not keen on taking pills. He asks about the evidence of benefits of antibiotics, and what the risks are if he declines to take them?

Where to start?
Once again, we try eTG complete, this time searching for 'bites'.

We see that dog bites have a lower risk of infection than cat bites and antibiotics may not be necessary, given that the wound does not involve joints or tendons. But the patient wants more details on whether antibiotics could provide benefit. For this, go to meta-analysis of controlled clinical trials; the Cochrane Library at
www.thecochranelibrary.org

Looking up the first record by Saconato produces a Cochrane systematic review, including a graph summarising the benefits of antibiotics according to the type of animal that inflicted the bite.

The graph shows that a number of trials of prophylactic antibiotics have been conducted on dog bites, albeit with small sample groups. No trial produced a statistically significant result alone (as shown by the 95 per cent confidence bars straddling an odds ratio of 1) nor was a statistically significant result produced when all trials were analysed together ($p = 0.6$).

If you find this graph a little complex, you can follow links to the abstract or synopsis of the review. There the author concludes there is no good evidence that prophylactic antibiotics for dog bites help to prevent infection, with the possible exception of bites on the back of the hand.

We can reassure the patient on the basis of the best available evidence that refusing to take antibiotics is unlikely to affect his chance of infection and that cleaning, debridement and irrigating the wound is currently recommended best practice. We should also check his tetanus immunisation status.

Summary

The case studies demonstrate how to use electronic knowledge resources to answer clinical problems in a timely manner and engage the patient in management decisions. Internet searches will find answers from a variety of sources. Use authoritative, distilled resources (Figure 4.1) before resorting to lower levels of evidence.

Use this chapter when practising searches of electronic resources. It will help you to:

- know when to use the Internet for finding answers to clinical queries
- ask a well-built (structured) clinical question
- know which sites are likely to provide relevant search results
- know how to search websites
- judge the relevance and quality of the information
- use this information in your clinical practice.

Computer security and general practice

05

Computer security in general practice is vital to ensure your business runs efficiently and to maintain the integrity of the electronic health records.

CONTENTS

When you have completed this chapter, you will be able to:

- appreciate the importance of computer security in your practice

- assess IT security risks in your practice

- design an IT security policies and procedures manual for your practice that covers the following issues:
  - practice security coordination
  - data access and passwords
  - disaster recovery
  - consulting room and front desk security
  - backups
  - viruses
  - firewalls
  - network maintenance
  - secure electronic communication

- list the roles and responsibilities of practice staff to support IT security

- identify the training needs and implement a training program, so that practice staff can competently perform their IT security tasks

- implement a schedule for the review of IT security procedures at specific intervals

- test, and review at specific intervals, a disaster recovery plan

- have increased confidence in the IT security procedures in your practice.

Introduction

Why do you need to think about computer security? Without it, your practice may experience costly down time in business operations or risk the loss of patient health information, making medical care more difficult and prone to errors.

The information in your electronic medical records is the most valuable component of your practice's computer system, and the most expensive to replace. You need to take all possible steps to protect it.

You won't need a high degree of technical knowledge to secure data, but you will need to understand the importance of computer security to your practice.

This chapter is intended as a resource to help you to establish and maintain computer security. It is not a technical guide. The chapter addresses aspects of accessibility, integrity and confidentiality and should help you to understand the main security risks likely to affect your practice.

The chapter is divided into two sections:
• organisational issues
• technical issues.

Computer security depends as much on people and what they do as it does on technical issues. Good communication and basic training for GPs and all practice staff is essential. For this reason, we discuss the organisational issues before the technical ones.

Organisational issues

WHO LOOKS AFTER COMPUTER SECURITY?

Your practice needs to be prepared for the inevitable computer crash. Ideally, your practice should have an IT security coordinator. This is not a technical 'fix it' person but someone responsible for overseeing computer security in the practice. This can be any person in the practice, and more than one person can share the responsibility. Quite likely they will be the person or persons responsible for computer issues in general.

The IT security coordinator ensures that:
• the practice adheres to an IT security policies and procedures manual
• staff members are trained
• staff understand their roles and responsibilities in relation to computer security
• the asset register (i.e. the list of all hardware and software) is up-to-date
• all operating manuals, installation disks and protocols are catalogued and securely stored
• there is a policy on staff access to computer data and systems
• the application for, storage and use of digital certificates, and training for practice staff on the use of encryption is coordinated
• staff know how and when to seek the advice of an IT technical support person.

For an example of an IT security coordinator role description see Figure 5.1. This role will vary from practice to practice, depending on the IT skills and interest of staff and the availability of technical support. Any member of staff can fill this role and some of the tasks can be shared. Modify this role to suit your purposes.

FIGURE 5.1 PRACTICE COMPUTER SECURITY COORDINATOR ROLE DESCRIPTION

General characteristics

This position suits someone who is enthusiastic about computers. They do not need advanced technical knowledge, although they should be reasonably comfortable with monitoring basic operating systems and relevant application software.

They must have management skills and be able to develop computer security policies in consultation with others in the practice. They may also be a general computer security coordinator for the practice.

Tasks

The computer security coordinator will:

- oversee the development of documented IT security policies and procedures
- oversee the development of a disaster recovery plan
- test disaster recovery procedures at specified intervals
- revise the disaster recovery plan at specified intervals
- keep an IT assets register (hardware, software, manuals and technical support)
- ensure there is an access control policy in place
- ensure staff are aware of the importance of maintaining password security
- ensure screensavers are in place
- establish a routine backup procedure
- test restoration of data at specified intervals
- install antivirus software on all computers and ensure virus definitions are updated daily
- install firewalls, seeking technical advice where required
- ensure computers, especially the server, are adequately maintained
- ensure the computer system can deal with fluctuations in the power supply
- investigate appropriate means of encrypting confidential information prior to electronic transfer
- coordinate the application for, use and storage of digital certificates and ensure the practice understands the use of encryption
- arrange computer security training for members of the practice.

REMEMBER!

You need to provide training for the security coordinator and review their role each year.

WHAT SHOULD BE IN THE COMPUTER SECURITY MANUAL?

Your practice may already have a policies and procedures manual, especially if you have completed practice accreditation. Make sure it includes the policies and procedures for computer security, such as:

- roles and responsibilities of all practice staff, in particular the role of the IT security coordinator

- a disaster recovery plan to keep the practice functioning when the computer system fails
- access rights (via passwords) to various levels of the clinical and practice management software
- an IT assets register of hardware, software and support services
- other aspects of computer security covered in this guideline.

The manual should contain phone numbers of software suppliers, details about operating systems and clarification of staff roles. The manual is also a tool to encourage you to think about your computer needs in terms of both human resource management and financial cost.

A computer security policies and procedures manual may sound like a lot of work, but it will help you clarify the issues in this chapter as they relate to your practice. It is important to continually review and update the manual as required.

You don't have to start from scratch. Download the template version of a computer security policies and procedures manual from the GPCG website at **www.gpcg.org.au**. Figure 5.2 also gives some guidelines as to what this manual should contain.

FIGURE 5.2 COMPUTER SECURITY POLICIES AND PROCEDURES GUIDELINES

Practice computer security coordinator
Your practice should appoint a computer security coordinator, whose role is defined and acknowledged by the practice (see Figure 5.1). The responsibilities of other staff should also be defined to determine the level of access to each system.

The computer security coordinator, who may be the general IT coordinator as well, should make sure staff are aware of the principles of computer security and are appropriately trained.

Disaster recovery plan
Your disaster recovery plan should:
- cover the critical functions of the practice so it can continue without major disruption or risk to the patients and staff
- contain the information necessary for returning the practice to its normal state.
  The plan will involve the creation of an asset register documenting:
- all hardware and software owned and used by the practice
- where the computer disks and manuals are stored
- who to phone for technical support and other assistance.

Maintain a log of faults as they occur. This helps in dealing with a range of minor and serious computer problems (see Figure 5.3).

(cont. overleaf)

FIGURE 5.2 COMPUTER SECURITY POLICIES AND PROCEDURES GUIDELINES (*cont'd*)

Backups

Document all details of the backup and recovery procedures. The backup procedure is a key component of the disaster recovery plan. Ensure backup media are taken off-site when the practice is closed. Record which members of staff perform the backups and automate as much of the procedure as possible (see Figure 5.3).

Internet and email

Provide a clear statement of the dos and don'ts regarding staff use of email and the Internet at the practice (see 'What should my Internet and email policies and procedures be?').

System access

Provide access to systems according to the responsibilities outlined in the role descriptions. Each staff member should create his or her own secure password/s. The system administrator's password should never be divulged to unauthorised persons.

Consulting room and front desk security

Document the practice policy on the use of screensavers and other precautions (such as the positioning of the monitors) to prevent unauthorised viewing of patient records and other confidential information.

Virus checking

Document virus-checking software and procedures (see Table 5.1).

Firewalls

Provide details of firewall hardware and software and their related procedures.

Maintenance

Computer maintenance is an aspect of core business. Document details of routine computer maintenance, including hard disk clean-ups and the physical security of the network.

Secure electronic communication

Record the practice policy on electronic communication of patient records and other confidential information. This involves authentication, encryption and associated procedures.

REMEMBER!

Write down computer security policies and procedures and ensure staff are clear about their responsibilities regarding IT security.

WHO SHOULD HAVE ACCESS TO DATA STORED ON THE COMPUTER?

Your practice must comply with national privacy principles. Data security helps to ensure the privacy of patient data and compliance with these principles.

Access to sensitive financial or clinical information should be on a need-to-know basis. Work out who can have access to what information. For example, what information should the receptionists or medical assistants be able to view? Restricted access also protects the practice against the misuse of financial data, and lessens the risk of accidental change or deletion.

Make sure each staff member has their own password to allow appropriate access to the operating system, application software and files within software, and email. Don't share passwords. There may be a high level of trust in your practice but it is not appropriate for your receptionist—or anyone else—to know your password and open your clinical software program each morning.

REMEMBER!

Your computer security policies and procedures should spell out appropriate levels of access for each staff member. Keep passwords secure and consider changing them periodically.

WHAT HAPPENS IF THE SYSTEM CRASHES?

Disasters can and do happen. When the computer system fails ('crashes'), be prepared! A disaster recovery plan outlines how your practice will continue to function in such an event.

When the computer system fails, you will still need to:
- make appointments for patients
- issue patients with invoices and receipts
- provide adequate clinical care.

You will need to know who to phone for technical advice about getting your system up and running again and to help retrieve data from backups (see the section on backups later in this chapter for information on this essential component of your recovery plan).

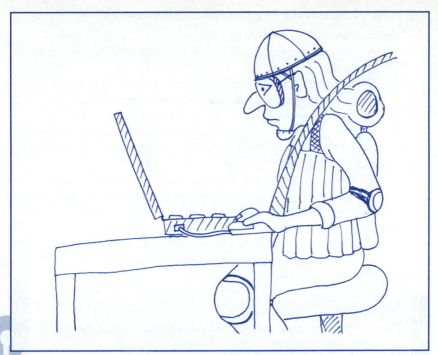

Always take precautions against system crashes

A disaster recovery plan will help to minimise disruption, the risk to the business, and the risk and inconvenience to patients. Your plan must define the critical functions managed by computers in your practice and outline any additional staff roles while the crash is active. The aim is for the practice to continue without major disruption to the patients and staff, thus ensuring no patient is put at risk. The plan should also contain procedures for returning the practice to its normal state following a system failure (you can download a template from the GPCG website at **www.gpcg.org.au**).

The recovery plan should outline:
• who phones for technical support
• who reinstalls the operating and application software
• who reloads the data
• what the practice needs to do to keep functioning in the meantime.

The plan should be reviewed periodically (e.g. annually), or when part of the plan changes, such as the backup media or procedure. Figure 5.3 outlines how you should approach disaster recovery.

FIGURE 5.3 DISASTER RECOVERY

Prepare a disaster recovery plan

Make a list of the critical practice functions, for example:

- making appointments
- providing adequate clinical care
- billing patients.

Discuss with staff how each of these is to be handled in the case of a disaster and how the switch to a paper-based system will occur.

Decide on who has overall charge of the recovery, and who is responsible for each function.

Create an asset register

This will consist of:

- hardware and software details, including their location within the practice
- network information
- the names and contact details of technical support personnel.

Create a fault logbook

Document in a logbook all computer faults, errors or full-blown disasters as they occur so the practice can learn how to combat future disasters. The log could include details of incidents such as:

- a virus on the system
- failure of the server
- failure of a computer to boot up
- failure of an individual computer or network component
- failure to connect to the Internet.

Coordinating the disaster recovery

The computer security coordinator should document the disaster recovery procedure step by step:

- first put in place the disaster recovery plan for administrative and clinical functions of the practice
- make a rapid and provisional investigation of what caused the crash
- contact technical support.

Implementing the restoration plan

Decide on who will be involved. The practice's administrative (appointment and billing) and clinical functions will need to be re-established before the computer restoration process commences. Locate the most recent backup and undertake an appropriate restoration (either complete or partial software and/or hardware replacement).

Reflecting after recovery

Review the disaster. What led to it? How did you restore function? How could you prevent it happening again? How could you refine the process?

Set aside some time to have a disaster practice run—a bit like a fire drill. Discuss with staff what each person will do in the event of the computer system crashing.

HOW DO I ENSURE PATIENT CONFIDENTIALITY?

Patients have the right to expect the privacy and confidentiality of their medical records be maintained. Be careful patients don't accidentally see another patient's health records during a consultation, or confidential financial information on computer screens at the reception desk. Consider each of the following techniques for maintaining privacy and choose those which suit your practice.

- Ensure staff maintain appropriate confidentiality of information on computer screens.
- Position screens so patients cannot see them.
- Use screensavers that appear with minimal delay.
- Use desktop shortcuts that turn on screensavers immediately.
- Use function keys that instantly clear the screen.

Technical issues

WHY DO I NEED TO KEEP COPIES OF FILES?

Backups are an important—if not the most important—IT security measure. The more dependent we become on computers, the higher the priority for backups.

Data can be lost through human error, or software or hardware problems. Loss of financial data can be costly, and the loss of clinical data can waste a significant amount of time. If a patient's previous medical conditions or drug allergies are recorded only in electronic form, then the loss of that information could put the patient at risk. Quality backups are also a useful medicolegal defence, providing an unaltered record of events at a particular time.

It is critical to backup all practice data on a regular basis. Restoration of data is part of your disaster recovery plan.

You need to know:

- the practice's backup procedure
- the backup media and software the practice uses
- how the practice restores the backup data.

The backup process should be as automated as possible. Ask your IT technical support person for advice.

HOW DO I ENSURE THAT DATA IS COPIED AND STORED?

Ensure your practice:
- backs up data daily
- stores backups off-site
- tests the backup procedure regularly (by performing and verifying a restoration of data)
- includes the backup procedure in a documented disaster recovery plan.

REMEMBER!

A backup is one of the most important aspects of a disaster recovery plan. Make sure you check your backup, and know how to reinstall your software programs as well as your data files.

HOW DO I PROTECT AGAINST VIRUSES AND OTHER THREATS?

Viruses (and the related worms, Trojans and other malicious codes) are programs that cause varying degrees of havoc in computer systems, including system slowdown and failure. This can have a major impact on your practice, especially if financial data is lost or altered.

Viruses can clog up the network and damage the reputation of the practice if the virus spreads through its electronic address books. Viruses can be 'caught' or transmitted:
- while communicating electronically via email or the Internet
- via floppy disks, CD-ROMs and other portable media.

The more time you spend on the Internet, the more likely you are to download a virus. Permanent connection via broadband increases this risk.

The following steps will help minimise the risks of virus infection:
- Have processes and programs in place to minimise the risk of downloading viruses from the Internet or introducing them from portable media brought in from outside the practice (make sure your software will not increase the risk of infection).
- Train staff in antiviral measures, as documented in the policies and procedures manual.
- Install antivirus software on all computers.
- Update antivirus software daily—you can adjust your settings so this will occur automatically.
- Perform a manual virus check. Some antivirus software can be set to automatically scan the hard disks of each computer in your practice at scheduled times (e.g. early each morning, when nobody is using the system). This will help to minimise the risk of infection to your system.

Other potential threats are spyware and spam. Spyware refers to programs that download themselves onto your computer while you are viewing a webpage. They can transmit information about your computer use to other sites. Spam is nuisance email. Spam and spyware are annoying and potentially threatening, as they can lead to inadvertent broadcasting of confidential information. Refer to the next section for procedures for minimising these risks.

WHAT SHOULD MY INTERNET AND EMAIL POLICIES AND PROCEDURES BE?

It is important to have a policy for staff regarding the use of the Internet and email. Make staff aware:

- of the need to maintain reasonable private use of email and the Internet during office hours (i.e. use that does not interfere with work efficiency)
- that viewing some websites during work time is inappropriate (e.g. pornographic or other sites that may cause offence)
- that it is not permitted to send email that might be construed as offensive or sexually harassing.

Make a statement to patients, such as:

Individual medical advice cannot be provided via email; all electronic data are subjected to privacy principles and no confidential information is to be transmitted without encryption.

This can be provided either on the practice website or in an information brochure.

Table 5.1 lists guidelines for the procedures you should have in place for using the Internet and email in your practice.

TABLE 5.1 PROCEDURES FOR INTERNET AND EMAIL USE	
Area of concern	Procedures
Protection against viruses	• Install and use antivirus software.
	• Keep this software active at all times.
	• Keep the software up-to-date using automatic updates. Periodically, check manually that it is up-to-date.
	• Apply patches to operating and application programs according to technical advice.
	• Do not download or open an email attachment if the sender is not personally known to you.
	• Do not open unexpected email, even from people known to you, as a virus may have spread this.
	• Do not open *.exe or *.bat attachments or other executable programs.
	• Use an antivirus mail filter to screen email prior to downloading.
	• Do not use the preview window in your email program as this automatically opens your email when you click on the header.
	• Save attachments and check for viruses before opening or executing them.
	• Do not run programs directly from websites. Download files and check them for viruses before running them.
	• Set and enable security settings in your Internet browser to medium or high.

	• Consider using Internet browsers and email programs that are more secure than some of the more frequently used versions.
	• Do not load software from floppy disks, CDs or USB memory sticks without first checking them for viruses (or gaining the consent of the security or systems coordinator).
Protection against theft of information	• Do not provide confidential information by email; only do so via the Internet when appropriate and when the site displays a security lock on the task bar.
	• Use a second, non-critical email address when registering personal details where you are not completely sure of the site's security.
	• Protect your email password.
Protection against hackers	• Install hardware and/or software firewalls between computers and the Internet (following technical advice). (If it's a software firewall, ensure everyone in the practice knows how to use it.)
	• Ask the technical support person to test the firewall periodically and update it as required.
	• If using a wireless network, seek technical advice on how to prevent others from hacking into your practice's network.
Protection against spam	• Do not reply to spam mail.
	• Never try to unsubscribe from spam sites—this merely confirms the existence of your email address.
	• Remain eternally vigilant: do not provide confidential information to an email (especially by return email), no matter how credible the sender's email seems (e.g. emails that look as though they originate from your bank).
	• Consider using a spam-filtering program.
Protection against spyware	• Learn how to recognise (and delete) spyware.
	• Don't accept certificates or downloads from suspect sites.
	• Consider installing antispyware software.
Encryption of patient information	• Do not send patient information or other confidential data by email unless you are using encryption, and it is appropriate to do so.
	• Encrypted files are not automatically checked for viruses. They have to be saved, decrypted and then scanned for viruses before being opened.
Backing up email and Internet favourites or bookmarks	• If you rely on information held in your email program, ensure it is backed up with the rest of your data.
	• If you have a useful list of Internet favourites or bookmarks make a backup of the list.

HOW CAN I KEEP HACKERS OUT OF MY COMPUTER SYSTEM?

There is no such thing as a foolproof system. Most people who spend significant amounts of time on the Internet will be aware that intrusions can occur with incredible frequency—perhaps several times an hour.

The best way to prevent unauthorised access to your practice computer system is to install a firewall. Firewalls are devices that block unauthorised access to your computer system. A firewall will help to prevent your system being identified by programs that scan the Internet looking for unprotected computers.

Firewalls can take the form of a hardware or software device. The most effective method is to install a hardware firewall. This acts as a protective device between the practice computer system and the Internet, preventing unauthorised access to or transfer of patient data. If you install a software firewall, ensure everyone in the practice knows how to use it.

Ask your technical support person for advice on the best options for your system. They should also regularly test and update your firewall. If you are using a wireless network, seek technical advice on how to prevent others with similarly equipped computers hacking into your practice's network.

REMEMBER!

Firewalls are essential for the long-term preservation of data and can help prevent patient information from inadvertently appearing on the Internet. They are as necessary as antivirus protection.

Make sure you test any hardware or software firewalls you install.

HOW DO I MAINTAIN MY COMPUTER AND NETWORK?

Regular computer and network maintenance prevents breakdowns and the slowing down of systems. Maintenance means looking after the equipment and the software. You should consider:

- how to keep your computer programs running efficiently
- physical protection of the computer, for example against theft
- protection against environmental damage such as heat, water and dust.

Computers are more likely to crash if they don't have enough free space on their hard drives. Install and maintain software according to the vendor's guidelines. Seek technical advice on how to keep your computer functioning most efficiently.

An uninterruptible power supply (UPS) can help to protect against the loss of data during a blackout. A UPS contains batteries to enable computers to shut down smoothly during a power cut. Install a UPS to the server at the very least. Simple surge protectors on other workstations will probably suffice.

A prolonged blackout constitutes an IT disaster. The only solution in such an occurrence is to use an electric generator, but this is usually too expensive for small businesses. Ask your technical support person if you should use more affordable power-saving techniques.

To prevent breakdowns, you should regularly:

- download operating system and other program patches (updates and repairs)
- run a program that cleans up file system errors and temporary files
- run a defragmentation utility program to increase available memory in your computer system
- update software
- keep liquids away from the keyboard and computer.

HOW CAN I MAKE MY ELECTRONIC COMMUNICATION SECURE?

You can protect sensitive electronic communication by encryption and
authentication:

- Encryption means that, with a simple click, your email is electronically
  scrambled and cannot be read until it is decrypted. Unless your
  practice has access to encryption, it is best not to send confidential
  data via email or the Internet.
- Authentication means you can confirm the identity of the sender by
  using electronic keys (i.e. identifying code).

Digital encryption services are available from a number of sources,
some at no cost. For example, the Australian Department of Health and
Ageing provides free digital encryption services to health care agencies,
including GPs. The system is called Public Key Infrastructure (PKI) which
is really a combination of policies, procedures and technology which
allows users to securely transfer information between computers. The
principles of PKI are similar to other forms of encryption systems in use.

There are many versions of PKI, and the Australian Government has
implemented one version which includes a health sector directory (i.e. a
list of people) and a PKI certificate infrastructure. Details about PKI are
available by going to **www.medicareaustralia.gov.au/providers/index.htm**
and searching for PKI.

PKI enables you to send a file to someone, and know that he or she is
the only person who can open it. You can also receive a file, confident it
has been sent to you securely.

In particular, with PKI, you know:

- who sent the message (authentication)
- that the content has not been altered between sender and receiver (integrity)
- that the sender cannot deny that he or she sent you the message (non-
  repudiation), and
- that only you, the intended receiver, can open the message.

PKI therefore allows data to be both encrypted and digitally 'signed',
the latter carrying the same legal value as a written signature. It achieves
this through the use of software, such as email programs, and
'certificates'. A digital certificate is an electronic document used to verify
the identity of a user. The certificate contains your name, a serial number,
the digital signature of the certificate-issuing authority (which is the Health
eSignature Authority, or HeSA, in the Australian system), and a copy of
the certificate holder's public 'key' (as explained below).

HeSA, which is known as a 'trusted third party' in PKI-talk, issues two digital certificates and two sets of keys (i.e. public and private key pairs, one pair for encryption and one for signing) to approved applicants. The keys, which are simply a large set of random numbers, are the basis of a system of cryptography. A public key is known to everyone and a private or secret key is known only to the recipient of the message. When Alice wants to send a secure message to Bob, she uses Bob's public key to *encrypt* the message. Bob then uses his private key to *decrypt* it.

An important element to the public key system is that the public and private keys are related in such a way that only the public key can be used to *encrypt* messages and only the corresponding private key can be used to decrypt them. Moreover, it is virtually impossible to deduce the private key if you know the public key.

The public/private key business can be quite confusing. It is worth going over it again in a slightly different way. Let us say that Alice wants to send Bob a secure email asking him if he will go out on a date with her. She signs her message with her secret private key and encrypts the message with Bob's public key which she has obtained from a public key directory (e.g. HeSA). Bob then receives the email and uses his private encryption key to *de*crypt the message. He also uses Alice's public signing key (obtained from the same directory) to confirm that the message really came from her.

In summary:
- the sender signs with a private signing key and encrypts with the other person's public encrypting key
- the receiver decrypts with their private encryption key and authenticates the sender by using the sender's public signing key.

Are you mixed up by the keys? Try this approach:
- Private keys generate digital signatures or decrypt encrypted information.
- Public keys encrypt information and verify the sender's digital signature. They are embedded in digital certificates and published in directories held by trusted third parties. Being public means that they can be used by other people who wish to send you information.

Of course, once people like Alice and Bob have obtained the required certificates and loaded the software, this process is very simple indeed. Email programs allow you to click on 'sign' and 'encrypt' and all the technical stuff happens in the background. It is virtually as easy as sending an ordinary email. The private key is located on a 'dongle', which is a small device which clicks into a USB port on the computer. This obviously needs to be connected when you are using PKI.

Certificates can be issued to organisations (location certificates) as well as individuals, and you will need to decide which one is easier to use in your practice. While a location certificate might appear to be easier, it will mean that a receiver of your message will know that it came from your practice, but theoretically, they cannot be sure it actually came from you.

05

PKI is very secure, but obtaining certificates can be quite a lengthy procedure—a bit like getting a bank loan. However, the main drawback is the encryption systems are not 'interoperable'; that is, you cannot use PKI at your end and communicate with someone who has another system such as PGP (Pretty Good Privacy) at their end. As we have seen in the section in Chapter 2 on interoperability, a lack of a uniform 'standard' way of doing things has been a major impediment to electronic connectivity among health care professionals.

Imagine if you could not communicate with someone who was using a mobile phone that belonged to a different company to your own; you would be pretty annoyed. But that is what happens with computer systems at this point in time.

If you do not use email regularly, and you don't feel that this is the right time to register for PKI, can you use email at all for transmitting clinical information? This is a matter of some controversy. Some would argue that if you wanted advice from a medical specialist on the management of a particular patient, you might be able to 'hide' the identity of the patient by withholding the name but using some other identifying phrase such as 'the patient with thyrotoxicosis that I referred to you last week'.

Perhaps this is a reasonable interim measure till a more universally adopted system is in place. It apparently has not been tested in the courts yet.

REMEMBER!

To respect the right of your patients to privacy, make sure your use of email is secure.

PRACTICAL EXERCISE

Consider these questions at your next practice meeting:

1 Who is your computer security coordinator?
2 What important information do you need to write down about your computer system?
3 What will you do if your computers suddenly crash in the middle of a consulting session? Write down a list of steps you will take to get your practice and then your computers up and running again.
4 How do you perform backups in your practice? Do they work? Have a review of the backup procedure in your practice.

(cont. overleaf)

5 Do all members of staff know how to minimise the risk of computer viruses? What would you do if your system became infected? Does your practice run an antispyware program, and do all staff know how to use it? Review the antivirus and antispyware programs on your computer.

- Do you have a firewall installed? Who in the practice knows about this? If you have a software firewall, do staff know how to use it?
- Who looks after your computer system? In particular, who ensures that the programs and systems are maintained from time to time, and appropriate update patches are installed?
- Have you considered encrypted email? Is it being used? What are the risks of sending unencrypted email?
- Is the practice computer system linked to your home computer? If so, what are the implications?

REMEMBER!

Computer security is not optional. Ignoring it will cause a problem one day.

Summary

A computer system crash could be a disaster for your practice. You need a suitable contingency plan, to minimise loss of business and patient care. This chapter has described the three components to computer security:

- availability – data can be found when needed
- integrity – data remains intact and accurate
- confidentiality – only authorised people are able to see the data.

Computer security comes with a financial cost. However, your practice computer system will fail one day, so it is imperative that you do not ignore security until it is too late.

- Seek expert, up-to-date technical advice.
- Assign a person in the practice to take responsibility for monitoring and addressing computer security issues.
- Ensure that everyone in the practice is aware of the importance of computer security.
- Produce policy and procedures manuals which help practice staff know what to do to keep your system secure.

Table 5.2 provides you with a checklist of computer security. The chapter describes each item in the checklist in more detail.

TABLE 5.2 COMPUTER SECURITY CHECKLIST

IT category	Tasks	Has this been implemented? (tick if yes)
1. Practice computer security coordinator	• Practice IT security coordinator's role description written.	☐
	• Practice IT security coordinator appointed.	☐
	• IT security training for coordinator provided.	☐
	• Security coordinator's role reviewed (at specified intervals).	☐
2. Practice IT security policies and procedures	• Person(s) (e.g. IT security coordinator) appointed to document (and revise) security policies and procedures (can be part of practice manual).	☐
	• IT security policies and procedures documented.	☐
	• IT security policies and procedures documentation reviewed (at specified intervals).	☐
	• Staff trained in IT security policies and procedures.	☐
3. Access control	• Staff policy developed on levels of electronic access to data and systems.	☐
	• Staff have created personal passwords to access appropriate level.	☐
	• Passwords are kept secure.	☐
	• Consideration given to changing passwords periodically.	☐
4. Disaster recovery plan	• Disaster recovery plan developed.	☐
	• Disaster recovery plan tested (at specified intervals).	☐
	• Disaster recovery plan updated (at specified intervals).	☐
5. Consulting room and 'front desk' security	• Practice aware of need to maintain appropriate confidentiality of information on computer screens.	☐
	• Screensavers or other automated privacy protection device enabled.	☐
6. Backups	• Backups of data done daily.	☐
	• Backups of data stored off-site.	☐
	• Backup procedure tested (by performing a restoration of data) at specified intervals.	☐
	• Backup procedure has been included in a documented disaster recovery plan.	☐
7. Viruses	• Antivirus software installed on all computers.	☐
	• Automatic updating of virus definitions enabled (daily if possible).	☐
	• Staff trained in antivirus measures as documented in policies and procedures manual.	☐
8. Firewalls	• Hardware and/or software firewalls installed.	☐
	• Hardware and/or software firewalls tested.	☐
9. Network maintenance	• Computer hardware and software maintained in optimal condition (includes physical security, efficient performance of computer programs, and program upgrades and patches).	☐
	• Uninterruptible Power Supply installed (to at least the server).	☐
10. Secure electronic communication	• Encryption systems considered.	☐
	• Encryption used for the electronic transfer of confidential information.	☐

Source: GPCG computer security project © February 2004

Promoting quality and safety in GP computing

The final chapter discusses what reasonable standards on computer use might be for the average GP. It also describes the educational roles for divisions of general practice and other professional bodies that could help improve GP computing skills. Finally, suggestions are made on how to encourage clinical software to match the needs of general practice.

CONTENTS

Introduction

This chapter has been written as a resource for organisations that are involved in continuing professional development and standard setting in general practice computing. It explains:

- what standards in GP computing are
- how divisions and other professional support organisations can help GPs attain these standards, and
- where GP computing might be heading to next.

The chapter is to be used in conjunction with the previous five chapters in this book. It will complement the educational programs that divisions and other professional bodies already have in place to promote GP computing.

The suggestions on GP computing do not assume that educators will have a background or qualifications in IM/IT, but they will have experience in delivering educational programs to GPs. This is an important role as there is very little formal training in the use of computers at either the undergraduate or postgraduate level. It seems that GPs are expected to learn about computers 'on the job'. That is not acceptable for other 'tools' that GPs use, such as the stethoscope, and it should not be for computing.

This chapter advocates the development of a comprehensive approach to standards in general practice computing, of which training is one component.

Setting standards for GP computing

WHAT COMPUTING STANDARDS SHOULD GPs HAVE?

Computing is a skill, and the areas in which GPs should become proficient can be defined and described. The RACGP's *Standards for general practices* 3rd edition (2005) has been developed to create benchmarks for quality in general practice. Several components of these 'standards' are relevant to GP computing, including: 'access to care' (standard 1.1); 'continuity of care' (standard 1.5); the 'content of patient health records' (standard 1.7); the 'management of health information' (standard 4.2); and 'facilities and access' (standard 5.1).

The RACGP standards form the basis for accreditation of general practices (see **www.racgp.org.au/standards**). They apply equally to paper-based and electronic records. It is helpful to consider these

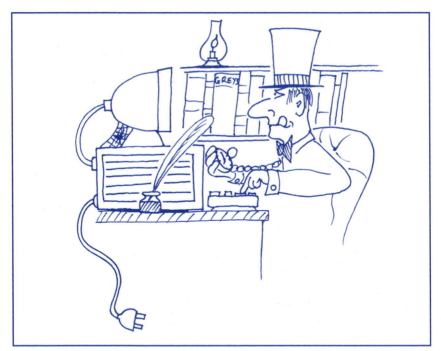

It's important to update your computer skills

standards in relation to quality and safety in GP computing, and that is why they are quoted at some length here.

The criteria which make up the College standards which are most relevant to the use of computers are:

- *Criterion 1.1.2 Telephone and electronic advice.* 'Patients of our practice are able to obtain advice or information related to their clinical care by telephone or electronic means where our GP(s) determine(s) that this is clinically safe and that a face-to-face consultation is unnecessary for that patient.'
- *Criterion 1.5.4 System for follow up of tests and results.* 'Our practice has a system for the follow up and review of tests and results.' The RACGP cautions that 'information technology can be a useful tool in follow up, however the current clinical information systems have limitations and may not provide sufficient safeguards to be relied on in all cases'.
- *Criterion 1.7.1 Patient health records.* 'For each patient we have an individual patient health record containing all clinical information held by our practice relating to that patient.'

- *Criterion 1.7.2 Health summaries.* 'Our practice incorporates health summaries into active patient health records.'
- *Criterion 1.7.3 Consultation notes.* 'Each of our patient health records contains sufficient information about each consultation to allow another doctor to carry on the management of the patient.'
- *Criterion 4.2.1 Confidentiality and privacy of health information.* 'Our practice has a systematic approach to managing the confidentiality and privacy of patient health information in our practice.'
- *Criterion 4.2.2 Information security.* 'The security of patient health information in our practice is maintained.'
- *Criterion 4.2.3 Transfer of patient health information.* 'On request by the patient, our practice transfers a summary or a copy of the patient health record to the patient, another medical practitioner, health service provider or health service.'
- *Criterion 4.2.4 Retention and destruction of patient health information.* 'Our practice has a system for the retention of—and any destruction of—patient health information.'
- *Criterion 5.1.1 Practice facilities.* 'Our practice facilities are appropriate for a safe and effective working environment for patients, staff and GPs.' This includes the practice having 'the capability for electronic communication by facsimile or email'.

These criteria have been quoted in some detail as they show that it is possible to define standards for GP computing, and their adoption can be measured. The measurement usually consists of a report by a 'surveyor' that a particular procedure is being followed to adopt the standard.

The Australian Government's 'Practice Incentives Program' ('the PIP') also stipulates certain criteria for GPs to obtain financial subsidies. In broad terms, the IT criteria are:

- *Tier 1: Basic.* The practice maintains electronic patient records, which include clinical data on allergies/sensitivities for the majority of active patients. In addition, the practice implements appropriate information security measures (e.g. virus protection, firewall, backup and recovery, access control and practice procedures/processes to support/maintain appropriate information security). The practice also uses appropriate security (e.g. encryption systems) when patient information and/or clinical data are transferred electronically.
- *Tier 2: Enhanced.* The practice qualifies for Tier 1 and uses electronic patient records to record and store clinical information on patients, including current and past major diagnoses and current medications for the majority of active patients.

'Broadband for Health' is a $60 million Australian Government program which helps provide broadband Internet access to GPs, Aboriginal Community Controlled Health Services (ACCHS) and community pharmacies nationwide. For GPs to obtain the subsidy, the government has requested information on their adherence to computer security guidelines which are based on the GPCG guidelines. These are referred to in Chapter 5.

It is therefore apparent that both the RACGP and government have indicated that GP computing should meet certain standards for the sake of patient safety and better-quality care.

A list of suggested standards which a 'computo-competent' GP should possess is presented in Figure 6.1. It could form the basis for a certificate in general practice computing in the future.

This list refers to the computer skills which each GP should have. In addition, one or more GPs within a practice, or non-GP staff, will need other computer skills. These include being able to liaise with IT technicians in the set up and maintenance of a practice-wide computer system.

There are four main areas of minimum skills a GP should possess when they sit down at their consulting desk:
• general computer tasks
• clinical software
• email and Internet
• security and privacy of electronic data.

The European Computer Driving Licence (see **www.ecdl.nhs.uk**) is a standard for general computer tasks, and has been applied to medical practitioners. The licence can be obtained after doing seven learning modules designed to give basic IT skills (i.e. basic IT concepts, using the computer and managing files, word processing, spreadsheets, databases, presentations, and information and communication). Although some of these skills arguably go beyond what is required in the clinical setting alone, the concept of a defined set of computer skills for doctors seems a good one.

Many GPs use a hybrid of paper-based and electronic medical records. The list of skills presented in Figure 6.1 assumes that GPs have made the transition to the latter. If you have not arrived at the point where all of your medical records are on the computer, then you might like to modify the list. It is only a guide, and there will no doubt be some disagreement on what are 'essential' skills and what are useful but not vital.

FIGURE 6.1 SKILLS FOR THE 'COMPUTO-COMPETENT' GP

The average GP should know the following:

A. FOR GENERAL USE OF THE COMPUTER, HOW TO:

1. turn on his or her workstation computer
2. use the keyboard and mouse
3. load from or connect a CD, DVD, floppy disk or USB memory stick
4. manage basic screen elements such as using a taskbar or dialog box
5. manage files and folders, including using file names, saving and opening files and printing documents
6. start up and log in to practice management and clinical software programs from the desktop
7. view the 'waiting room' within practice management software
8. 'call in' the next patient from the 'waiting room', thereby opening a clinical file.

B. FOR CLINICAL SOFTWARE, HOW TO:

9. create an accurate past medical history list for the majority of one's patients
10. prescribe safely; that is, appropriate use of drug interaction warnings, using a method to check appropriate drug doses (e.g. in children or patients with renal impairment), knowing where to look up prescribing information
11. record drug allergies for most patients
12. record smoking, alcohol and family history for the majority of patients
13. enter sufficient clinical information into the medical record so that another doctor is able to use them
14. enter measurements in the appropriate fields (e.g. blood pressure, height, weight)
15. develop a system for managing pathology and radiology results that minimises the risk of missing a significant test, or failing to act on an abnormal result
16. record immunisations
17. use a reminder system (sometimes called an 'action list'); that is, a system in which you can set up a computer prompt which is activated the next time your patient returns
18. manage a recall system; that is, add patients to a recall list and establish a process for recalling a patient on the due date
19. use templates for a variety of tasks, including chronic disease management
20. write referral letters with relevant clinical information included
21. conduct database searches (e.g. for patients with type 2 diabetes)
22. add some structure to the progress notes (e.g. entering a 'reason for visit' or 'diagnosis', as appropriate)
23. use shortcuts (e.g. abbreviations which trigger the entry of previously defined text).

C. FOR EMAIL AND INTERNET, HOW TO:

24. send and receive email
25. use email securely (which might involve the use of encryption methods but also includes the safe viewing of attachments)
26. search for a website by either using a search engine or entering a web address (URL)

D. FOR KEEPING ELECTRONIC DATA SECURE AND PRIVATE, HOW TO:

27. use computer security guidelines to maintain the security of your electronic data, especially if you have an Internet connection (see Chapter 5 on computer security for guidelines on this)
28. use clinical records and email in a manner consistent with privacy principles, and which adheres to the reasonable expectations of patients in general.

Use the items in Figure 6.1 as a checklist to see what you currently know and what the gaps are in using your computer in your practice. Discuss this with your colleagues at a practice meeting, if appropriate, and work out how each of you can be supported to increase your computing skills. You could learn more about computing by 'show and tell' sessions with your colleagues in front of a computer or by obtaining advice and training from your local division of general practice.

ACCREDITATION: WHAT STANDARDS SHOULD CLINICAL SOFTWARE HAVE?

It is one thing to expect GPs to attain certain computing standards: what about the clinical software programs that GPs use? What reassurance do GPs have that their programs conform to safety standards (e.g. for drug interaction checking) or are reliable so that data is not lost during upgrades? Developing a regulatory framework for clinical software is a task which has proved quite daunting in the Australian setting. The purpose of such a framework is to establish a process for the accreditation of software.

The Australian Medical Association (see **www.ama.com.au** and follow the links to general practice and e-health under 'policy and issues') has recommended that a number of key issues be considered in establishing an accreditation framework:

- effective consultation with the software industry which not only sets out acceptable specifications but is financially viable
- defining technical specifications so that software is 'interoperable'
- defining functional specifications so that software performs according to the needs of the users (i.e. GPs)
- deciding on whether to accredit the software vendors or their products
- deciding on whether it is only feasible to regulate a process (i.e. the vendor has to demonstrate that their product uses an acceptable process to incorporate drug–drug interaction warnings), or whether it is possible to do 'laboratory' tests of programs (e.g. to see if drug–drug interactions really work)
- developing a mechanism for feedback from users which might indicate shortcomings in software (a bit like post-marketing surveillance of pharmaceutical products).

It would appear that such a regulatory body would need to be set up and funded by government, with professional, industry and consumer input. No wonder it has not yet seen the light of day!

An alternative approach could be for the RACGP and similar professional bodies to set up their own accreditation process. The RACGP would have a committee which is funded by fees paid by clinical software companies that wish to have their products accredited. The College would publish which software packages are accredited, and GPs would be encouraged to use only these. This should provide incentives for the vendors to comply. Guidelines for software accreditation indicate that software should:

- use a secure database (e.g. so that it does not lose data when the program is upgraded according to the vendor's instructions)
- be interoperable with other accredited clinical software (i.e. its data can be uploaded to another package)
- adopt functionalities that allow GPs to perform the tasks specified for the 'computo-competent' GP (Section B of Figure 6.1)
- provide clinically sound decision support by using a process of ensuring safety which is acceptable to the medical profession (e.g. by providing drug interactions based on government-approved prescribing information)
- be up-to-date with government legislation as it affects general practice (e.g. through the provision of appropriate templates to assist with chronic disease management)
- demonstrate increasing adherence to nationally accepted standards (technical and semantic).

As can be seen, this approach to accreditation involves the RACGP software accreditation committee being satisfied that the vendor has taken appropriate measures to ensure that their product is safe, useful and promotes quality in health care. It is 'process' accreditation. It is doable, although it should not be used by government as a substitute for a more rigorous system as has been applied to drugs and medical devices.

The approach in the United Kingdom has been to develop programs which seek to establish standards via IT systems and the individual GP (see **www.connectingforhealth.nhs.uk/**). The National Health Service (NHS) Connecting for Health is an agency of the Department of Health. Its primary role is to deliver new, integrated IT systems and services to help modernise the NHS and ensure care is centred on the patient.

The new computer systems and services will connect over 110 000 doctors, 390 000 nurses and 120 000 other health professionals.

There are several components to NHS Connecting for Health:

- The *NHS Care Records Service* with an individual electronic NHS Care Record for every patient in England, securely accessible by patients and those caring for them.

- The electronic booking service, *Choose and Book*, offering patients greater choice of hospitals or clinics and more convenience in the date and time of their appointment.
- *Electronic Prescription Service* to make prescribing and dispensing safer, easier and more convenient for patients.
- A new *National Network* providing IT infrastructure and broadband connectivity for the NHS so patient information can be shared between organisations.
- *NHSmail*, a central email and directory service for the NHS to enable staff to transfer patient information swiftly, securely and efficiently.
- *Picture Archiving and Communications Systems* to capture, store, display and distribute static and moving digital medical images, providing clearer X-rays and scans and faster, more accurate diagnosis.
- IT supporting GPs, including the *Quality Management and Analysis System*, support for the Quality and Outcomes Framework (QOF) and the system for *GP to GP record transfer*.

The Quality and Outcomes Framework (QOF) is part of the new General Medical Services contract for general practices, and was introduced on 1 April 2004. The QOF provides financial rewards to general practices for the provision of high quality care. It measures achievement against a scorecard of 146 indicators, plus three measures of depth of care.

The QOF comprises four domains:

- *Clinical.* Seventy-six indicators in eleven areas: coronary heart disease, left ventricular disease, stroke or transient ischaemic attack, hypertension, diabetes, chronic obstructive pulmonary disease, epilepsy, hypothyroidism, cancer, mental health and asthma.
- *Organisational.* Fifty-six indicators in five areas: records and information about patients, patient communication, education and training, practice management and medicine management.
- *Patient experience.* Four indicators in two areas: patient surveys and consultation length.
- *Additional services.* Ten indicators in four areas: cervical screening, child health surveillance, maternity services and contraceptive services.

Clinical software programs have to allow GPs to extract data which can be used to demonstrate compliance with the indicators. The English appear to prefer the 'top down' approach to establishing standards for clinical IT (see **www.rcgp.org.uk**, search for RCGP Curriculum Statement 4.2, and then follow the link to Information Management and Technology); this approach might be good if you believe that governments and professional organisations are capable of choosing the 'right' system!

Supporting standards: the role of divisions of general practice

WHAT IS THE HISTORY OF DIVISIONAL SUPPORT FOR COMPUTING IN GENERAL PRACTICE?

General practice computing has had a relatively rapid uptake from the late 1990s on. Chapter 1 outlines a number of reasons why this occurred. Part of the explanation lies with the support provided by the 'IT officer program' for divisions of general practice, which ran between 1999 and 2001. Divisions employed project officers with a variety of skills, ranging from those who could provide 'help desk' support through to those whose skills were more restricted to information management. Subsequently, divisions applied information management principles to their chronic disease management (CDM) and Enhanced Primary Care (EPC) programs, although the majority of divisions did not continue to employ specific IT officers.

In 2005, the Australian Divisions of General Practice (now called the Australian General Practice Network), a peak body for the Divisions Network, announced the formation of a program involving eleven Regional Health Information Management Officers (RHIMOs) who are based within each of the divisions' state-based organisations (SBOs).

These initiatives reinforce the ongoing importance of computing in general practice, and that GPs still need support to improve the standard of computing, especially for patient care. This section is written on the assumption that the Divisions Network will be one of the principal means by which GP education in computing is delivered. However, the educational strategies can be used by other professional organisations as well.

WHAT WOULD A GP COMPUTER EDUCATION SYLLABUS COVER?

The broad domains of GP computing which a divisional education program can consider are:
- general computing skills (e.g. use of the keyboard, skills in using common programs such as word processing, email and the Internet); these skills are not described in detail in this book which has a narrower emphasis on computing in general practice
- the consultation, including the use of computers that supports the GP–patient relationship, and privacy and other ethical and legal issues (Chapter 1)
- practice management (Chapter 2)
- clinical care (Chapter 3)

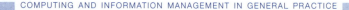

- the role of the practice, to support the optimal use of computers for patient management and business efficiency (Chapters 1 to 5)
- evidence-based medicine, including use of the Internet, evidenced-based guidelines and peer-reviewed electronic textbooks (Chapter 4)
- electronic data security (Chapter 5).

This book can be recommended as a resource by divisions for their computer education programs and should be seen as a complete package (see Table 6.1). It deals with principles that can be widely applied across most computer and medical software programs, although professional IT advice or software manuals might be needed to learn about particular applications.

TABLE 6.1 IM/IT TOPICS SUITABLE FOR A GP COMPUTER EDUCATION PROGRAM

Module	Details
Chapter 1—Computers, GPs and patients: issues in general practice	Contains three sections: optimal use of computers within the consultation; privacy and confidentiality of consumer health information; and legal issues. Provides an outline of what general practice staff need to know about: • the benefits of using computers in the consultation • making the most of computers in the consultation • privacy of health information • using and sharing health information • security of health information • using email in general practices • legal issues relating to the collection, use, storage and security of health information.
Chapter 2—Computers and practice management	Outlines key features of: • practice management software, including government incentives for businesses • hardware and networking issues • typing and basic computer skills • technological innovations (e.g. remote access).
Chapter 3—Computers and clinical care	Highlights the main features of clinical software, and how they can be used most effectively in clinical care. This includes: • recalls and reminders • the use of templates • progress notes (i.e. full electronic medical record).
Chapter 4—Electronic resources	Provides practical tips on finding a range of evidence-based electronic clinical resources. This includes: • clinical guidelines • peer-reviewed electronic textbooks • journal articles.
Chapter 5—Computer security	Provides a step-by-step guide through a range of IT risk categories and general practice based on the GPCG security guidelines. This includes: • human resources • backups and disaster recovery procedures.

The ability of division staff (or that of other professional organisations) to deliver a GP computer education program will vary and is dependent on the available skills, experience and resources.

Simply providing the training and information to general practice staff does not guarantee adoption within general practice. The training must:
- be relevant to the learner
- involve active rather than passive participation
- form part of a change in the management framework to encourage GPs and general practice staff to increase their use and understanding of IM/IT, in order to improve the quality of patient care and business efficiency.

Practices may not be interested in or ready to explore all five chapters. However, divisions can offer its educational messages over time.

There are a number of ways for divisions to deliver the educational program (see Table 6.2). It is designed for face-to-face delivery, but eventually it would be better if it were a web-based educational resource.

TABLE 6.2 DELIVERY OPTIONS FOR A GP COMPUTING EDUCATIONAL PROGRAM

Delivery method	Details
Practice visits	Divisional project officers conduct practice visits to assist GPs and other staff to adopt the minimum standards in IM/IT, as described in this book. This can be achieved through: • one-on-one education • group sessions.
Division workshops	Divisions offer IM/IT workshops to GPs and general practice staff, in which a small number of participants are guided through practical exercises on the computer. This would ideally take place in a computer lab, although if there are not enough computers, using a data projector is the next best option.
Divisional support for practices	Other support to practices could include: • written materials • telephone support • email bulletins.

The strategies used will depend on the resources available to divisions, as well as the willingness and ability of GPs and other general practice staff to participate in a particular format. For example, it may be easier and more convenient for a program officer to visit a practice than to have participants travel to a central location.

These issues affect other continuing professional development (CPD) activities, but IM/IT is best learned through a hands-on approach (i.e. on a computer). Few divisions will have ready access to computer education labs. Divisions might consider pooling some of their office computers to create an equivalent environment.

It is recommended that divisions map out a 1- to 2-year program that comprises the following elements:

- computers in the consultation
- administrative aspects of computers
- clinical aspects of computers
- using the Internet, and
- computer security.

Further information about such a program is provided in Table 6.1.

Future directions

Aspects of this book will need to be updated because GP computing is, as you know, a rapidly changing field. For example, electronic communication between health care providers has only just begun. The idea of a shared electronic health record held in cyberspace remains nothing much more than a pilot-tested dream at this stage, but who doubts that it will be developed, and fairly soon? Personal digital assistants, wireless connectivity from anywhere ... the list of exciting developments is endless.

However, whatever the current IT system, its optimal use by GPs should lead to better patient care and increased business efficiency. No matter where computers are heading, GPs need to keep up their computing skills in order to provide safe and good quality clinical care. There is no need to wait till the next IT 'breakthrough'.

Developments in IT provide challenges for a number of groups:

- for government—to develop standards in IT and help create ways of implementing them
- for the computer software industry—to adopt standards and make computer programs which meet GP's needs
- for the medical profession—to define the computer skills GPs should have, and assist in their uptake
- for GPs and their practices—to adopt 'best practice' in using computers.

Education in computing will remain an important aspect of meeting the challenge of IT in general practice. Divisions and other professional organisations have a major role to play in encouraging and supporting GPs to put their computers to optimal use.

The real challenge for groups such as divisions is for them to take a substantial interest in GP computer education when there are so many other programs to run. Divisions might be less inclined to pursue computing as an activity unless there is a reasonable demand to do so by

GPs. Without strong commitment from within a division, or with a 'we'll wait and see what the demand is' attitude, a computer education program is unlikely to get off the ground.

Likely drivers for GP training and education in computing will include IM/IT standards in practice accreditation, continuing government subsidies to GPs for meeting IM/IT criteria and support by the Divisions Network itself, for example via the RHIMO program. Demands for quality and safety in medicine also seem to be increasing from several quarters, and these are likely to have an impact on GP education in this field.

Summary

The lessons of the last few years suggest that GP computer education is a journey which has its stops and starts. However, the increasing computerisation of general practice, and its inevitable e-connectivity with other sections of the health care system, will make the need for a more formalised education program self-evident.

Quality and safety in computing will become increasingly important issues as electronic medical records become the norm. This means that there will need to be standards set for general practice computing as well as the clinical software that GPs use.

Glossary

ADSL Asymmetrical digital subscriber line. The most common broadband Internet system in Australia. It uses standard copper phone lines to carry the Internet signals, but operates separately from the telephone.

Backup (noun) The saved or backed up files. This may be in the form of a removable disk or tape, or to another system.

Backup (verb) To save a copy of your data and/or entire system so you can recover from catastrophes ranging from loss of some data to loss of the entire system, should they occur.

Broadband A 'fast' Internet connection. What speed is considered to be broadband differs around the world. In Australia we have very low expectations—a data transfer speed above 256 kilobytes per second is considered to be broadband. Common broadband access systems are ADSL, cable, satellite and wireless.

Cat 5 and Cat 5e The two standard types of (blue) networking cable.

Database A computer program enabling collection, storage and access to data in an organised manner. Also refers to the files associated with the program.

Ethernet The normal, wired networking standard.

File A collection of data stored on a computer. A file may be a single document or image or a series of related documents, such as a patient database.

Hard disk The primary storage system within a computer. It holds the operating system, software and data files. Hard disks inevitably fail on occasion, hence the need for backups.

Hardware Any physical part of the computer system. This includes the computer, monitor, keyboard and mouse as well as peripherals such as printers and modems.

ICT Information and communication technology.

IM Information management. The management of information according to its intended and potential uses. Available technological resources are a major consideration in IM.

Internet A worldwide communications system for transferring and accessing information. Most information on the Internet is free, but accessing the Internet itself usually costs money (see ISP).

ISP Internet service provider. The commercial company that provides you with access to the Internet. This can be via wired or wireless methods. The ISP usually provides email accounts as well.

IT Information technology. An all-encompassing term for computer systems.

LAN Local area network.

Licence A software program is usually only licensed for use on one computer. In some cases you can purchase extra licences to run the software on more than one computer. Licences may apply for the life of the product or only for a fixed period, such as one year. Updates may or may not be included in the purchase price.

Monitor The computer screen. Originally a television picture tube, now most commonly a thin, flat liquid crystal display panel such as those found in a notebook PC.

Mouse A hardware component allowing for simple and fast navigation of the computer system. If you've never used a PC you might wonder why you'd need a mouse. It's simply because a mouse will make you infinitely more productive. It takes little time to learn to use. Notebooks have an inbuilt pointing device (mouse substitute) but many users find it preferable to install a mouse.

Network (noun) A catch-all term to describe two or more computers or devices that are connected together using wired and/or wireless networking systems. The function of a network is to allow users and devices on the network to share resources such as files, storage, Internet access and printers. Basic networking capabilities are built in to all operating systems.

Network (verb) To connect two or more computers or computer devices together in such a way that more devices can be connected if required.

Network, client/server A network that uses one or more servers to provide services and control for multiple users.

Network, peer to peer A network of PCs that are connected together to share resources, but with no server.

Notebook Also known as 'laptop' PCs. A notebook is a portable PC with inbuilt screen, keyboard and pointing device, though all three may be replaced with plug-in versions. A notebook has a battery for portable use.

Operating system The foundation software that enables a PC to operate. Microsoft Windows is the most common operating system. The other two in common use by GPs are Mac OS X and Linux. The operating system usually includes basic applications, but any specialised applications must be bought separately (e.g. word processing).

Password A word or phrase that must be used in conjunction with a user name in order to access some systems and applications.

PC Personal computer. There are various names for the box that is the computer, such as central processing unit (CPU), system unit and tower.

PDA Personal digital assistant. A handheld PC.

Peripheral A device connected to the computer (e.g. printer, scanner, web camera).

Product activation Some software won't work (or won't work beyond a certain period) unless it is 'activated' by contacting the manufacturer. This is usually done over the Internet, but may be done by phone. The idea is to prevent unauthorised use of software. In general, a product may only be installed and used on one computer.

Product registration A system of letting the software manufacturer know who you are and that you're using the software. This may not be compulsory, but it helps keep the product up-to-date by allowing notifications of upgrades.

Seat One form of computer application licence. You might purchase three 'seats', which means that three different users will be able to use the application on three PCs concurrently. Some software is licensed by 'user', which means you must purchase a licence for each individual user.

Security A broad concept encompassing the physical and electronic security of your data and system. This includes antivirus, antispyware, firewalls, passwords, backup, physical security and more.

Server A computer that provides central resources and control for a network. In general it is not used as a workstation.

Software A set of instructions necessary to get the computer to perform a task. While some software applications are built into the operating system, you usually have to obtain extra software to get the computer to perform a specific job. Commercial software has specific rules about where and when it can be used. There are also various sorts of freeware and shareware that can be used more freely. The term 'package' is often used to describe a piece of software.

SQL Structured query language. A common database structure that allows users to create queries for retrieving data. In most cases the software package will deal with the database for you.

UPS Uninterruptible power supply. A device that sits between the mains power and devices such as a PC. It has a battery that generates a 240-volt supply when the mains power fails or momentarily drops out. This gives you enough time to save your files and shut the system down.

VoIP Voice over Internet Protocol. Commonly used to conduct Internet telephony or make phone calls via the Internet.

VPN Virtual private network. A system that allows a user to connect to a remote service via the Internet, but through a secure 'tunnel'. For instance, you could connect to your surgery from home or another office via VPN.

WiFi Wireless networking. Also known as the 802.11 family of standards.

Workstation A PC that is designed to be operated by a user (as distinct from a server).

Index